THIS KETO DIET JOURNAL BELONGS TO:

90 DAYS OF KETO

STARTING WEIGHT: **DAY 90 WEIGHT:**

1	2	3	4	5	6	7	8	9	10	**LBS LOST:** **INCHES LOST:**
11	12	13	14	15	16	17	18	19	20	**LBS LOST:** **INCHES LOST:**
21	22	23	24	25	26	27	28	29	30	**LBS LOST:** **INCHES LOST:**
31	32	33	34	35	36	37	38	39	40	**LBS LOST:** **INCHES LOST:**
41	42	43	44	45	46	47	48	49	50	**LBS LOST:** **INCHES LOST:**
51	52	53	54	55	56	57	58	59	60	**LBS LOST:** **INCHES LOST:**
61	62	63	64	65	66	67	68	69	70	**LBS LOST:** **INCHES LOST:**
71	72	73	74	75	76	77	78	79	80	**LBS LOST:** **INCHES LOST:**
81	82	83	84	85	86	87	88	89	90	**LBS LOST:** **INCHES LOST:**

TOTAL WEIGHT LOST: **TOTAL INCHES LOST:**

NOTES & REFLECTIONS:

KETO CHALLENGE START DATE

What you hope to achieve from doing Keto

Describe how you see yourself in six months

DATE	KETO HEALTH/WEIGHT LOSS ACTION PLAN	PERSONAL MILESTONES

MONTH BY MONTH PROGRESS QUICK VIEW

JANUARY

FEBRUARY

MARCH

APRIL

MAY

JUNE

JULY

AUGUST

SEPTEMBER

OCTOBER

NOVEMBER

DECEMBER

MILESTONES

NOTES & REFLECTIONS

KETO BEFORE & AFTER

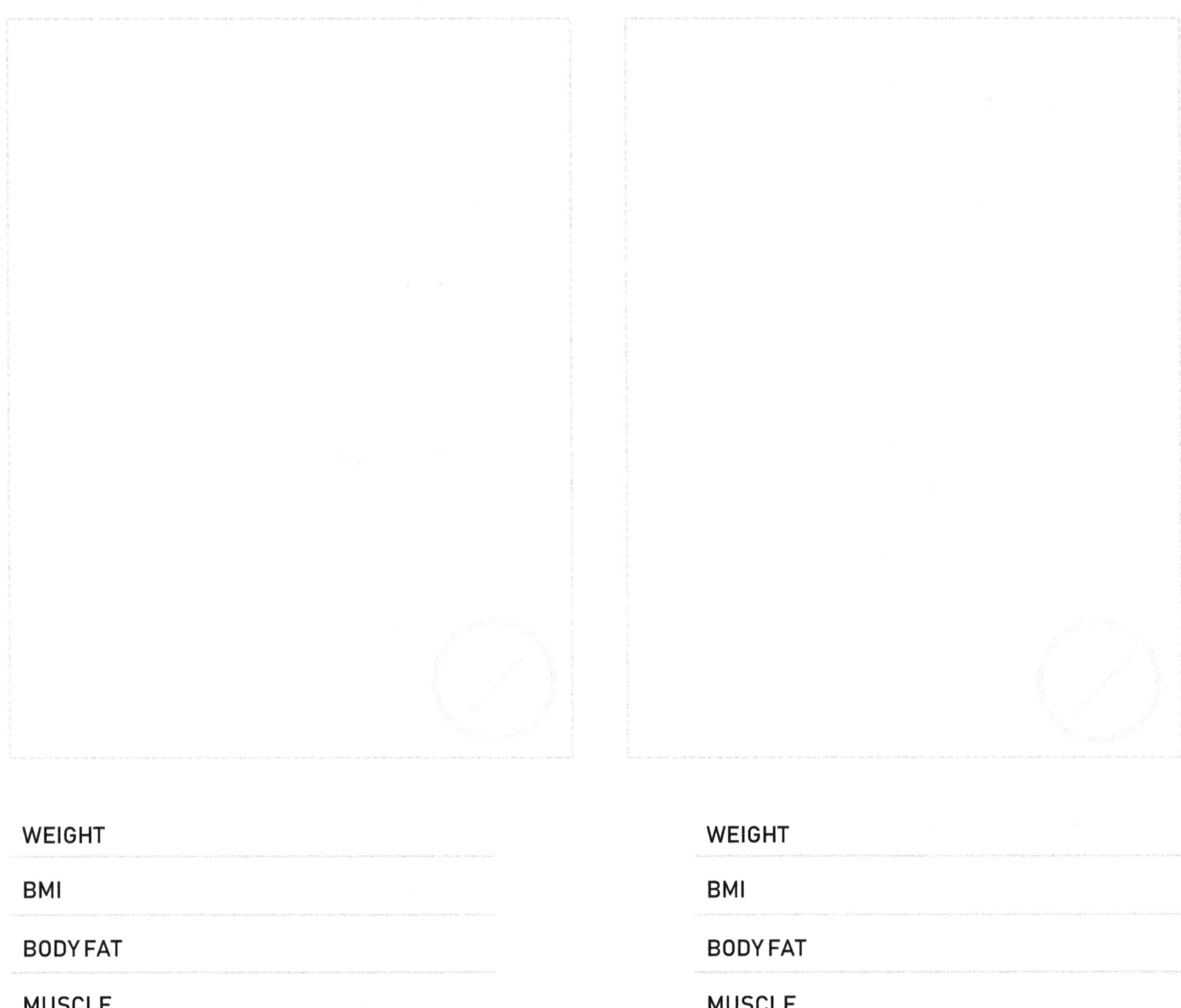

WEIGHT	WEIGHT
BMI	BMI
BODY FAT	BODY FAT
MUSCLE	MUSCLE
CHEST	CHEST
WAIST	WAIST
HIPS	HIPS
THIGHS	THIGHS
CALF	CALF
BICEP	BICEP
OTHER :	OTHER :
OTHER :	OTHER :

STARTING MEASUREMENTS

MONTHLY GOAL

DATE:

	CHEST				
	WAIST				
	SHOULDERS				
	UPPER ARM				
	FOREARM				
	CALF				
	WEIGHT				

TOTAL WEIGHT LOSS >>

KETO 15 CHALLENGE

1 CREATE A KETO JOURNAL AND DOCUMENT YOUR PROGRESS — COMPLETED ☐	**2** CHOOSE 7 KETO FRIENDLY RECIPES TO TRY — COMPLETED ☐	**3** CREATE A WEEKLY MEAL PLANNER — COMPLETED ☐
4 LOG EVERYTHING YOU EAT IN A WEIGHT LOSS APP — COMPLETED ☐	**5** PURCHASE A FOOD SCALE AND SPIRALIZER — COMPLETED ☐	**6** TRY BULLET PROOF COFFEE — COMPLETED ☐
7 WEIGH YOURSELF EVERY WEEK — COMPLETED ☐	**8** GO ALCOHOL FREE FOR ONE WEEK — COMPLETED ☐	**9** TRY A 12-HOUR INTERMITTENT FAST — COMPLETED ☐
10 CHECK AND LOG YOUR BODY MEASUREMENTS — COMPLETED ☐	**11** LIST ALL THE REASONS WHY KETO WILL WORK FOR YOU — COMPLETED ☐	**12** LEARN TO MAKE FAT BOMBS — COMPLETED ☐
13 MONITOR YOUR WATER INTAKE — COMPLETED ☐	**14** INCREASE YOUR HEALTHY FAT INTAKE — COMPLETED ☐	**15** TEST KETONE LEVELS USING STRIPS — COMPLETED ☐

KETOGENIC FOODS

MEATS	VEGGIES	VEGGIES	FRUITS
Beef	Avocado	Cucumber	Blackberries
Sausage	Asparagus	Chards	Cranberries
Bacon	Argula	Bell Peppers	Blueberries
Lamb	Broccoli	Green Beans	Lemon
Pork	Cauliflower	Collards	Lime
Veal	Brussel Sprouts	Mushrooms	Raspberries
Chicken/Turkey	Cabbage	Spinach	Strawberries
Eggs	Celery	Olives	Plantains (paleo)

DAIRY	CONDIMENTS	OILS & FATS	HERBS & SPICES
Cheese (all kinds)	Balsamic Vinegar	Avocado Oil	Garlic
Sour Cream	Beef/Chicken Broth	Butter	Salt & Pepper
Cream Cheese	Bonito Flakes	Coconut Butter	Oregano
Heavy Cream	Tartar Sauce (keto)	Duck Fat	Paprika
Greek Yogurt	Dijon Mustard	Lard/Ghee	Cumin
Almond Milk	Mayo	Nut Oils	Chili Pepper
Cashew Milk	Low Sugar Ketchup	Olive Oil	Basil
Coconut Cream	Pickles	Pork Rinds	Ginger

BAKING	FISH/SEAFOOD	DRINKS	MISC.
Almond Flour	Anchovy	Diet Soda (moderation)	Canned Tuna
Almond Meal	Haddock / Cod	Coffee	Pesto
Cashew Flour	Halibut	Tea	Soy Sauce
Oat Fiber	Crab/Lobster	Gatorade Zero	Aioli
Psyllium Husk	Mackerel	Protein Shake	Béarnaise
Whey Protein	Salmon	Club Soda	Vinaigrette
Flax meal	Tuna	Broth	Hot Sauce
Hazelnut Flour	Red Snapper	Coconut Water	Guacamole

NOTES:

LOW CARB GROCERY IDEAS

FRESH PRODUCE

Asparagus	Cauliflower	Onions
Avocado	Celery	Radishes
Bell Peppers	Cucumber	Salad Mix
Berries	Eggplant	Squash
Broccoli	Fennel	Tomatoes
Brussel Sprouts	Garlic	Bok Choi
Cabbage	Green Beans	Chives
Carrots	Mushrooms	Spinach

MEAT AND SEAFOOD

Bacon	Lamb	Fish
Beef	Pork	Crab
Bison	Rotisserie Chicken	Lobster
Chicken	Sausage	Scallops
Deli meat	Turkey	Shrimp
Ground Beef / Ground Turkey	Oyster	Mussels

DAIRY PRODUCTS

Butter	Eggs	Sour Cream
Cheese	Greek Yogurt, full fat	Ghee
Cream Cheese	Heavy Whipping Cream	Mayo

PANTRY ITEMS

Avocado oil	Tea/Coffee	Moon Cheese
Beef Jerky	Pork Rinds	Low Carb Protein Bars
Bone Broth	Mayonnaise	All Natural Peanut Butter
Tuna, Salmon (canned)	Low Carb Salad Dressing	Stevia
Coconut Butter	Olive oil, extra virgin	Almonds
Coconut Oil	Olives	Spices
Almond Milk	Sweeteners	Almond Flour

FROZEN / OTHER

KETO FRIENDLY FOODS

KETO FRIENDLY FOODS	NET CARBS	PROTEINS	FAT

FOODS TO EAT IN MODERATION	NET CARBS	PROTEINS	FAT

KETO FRIENDLY FOODS

KETO FRIENDLY FOODS	NET CARBS	PROTEINS	FAT

FOODS TO EAT IN MODERATION	NET CARBS	PROTEINS	FAT

KETO GO TO MEALS

BREAKFAST	LUNCH	DINNER	SNACKS
BREAKFAST	LUNCH	DINNER	SNACKS
BREAKFAST	LUNCH	DINNER	SNACKS
BREAKFAST	LUNCH	DINNER	SNACKS
BREAKFAST	LUNCH	DINNER	SNACKS
BREAKFAST	LUNCH	DINNER	SNACKS
BREAKFAST	LUNCH	DINNER	SNACKS

KETO RECIPE

RECIPE NAME:

Keto	Low Carb	Paleo	Vegetarian	Vegan	Dairy Free	Gluten Free
☐	☐	☐	☐	☐	☐	☐

QTY	INGREDIENTS	RECIPE INSTRUCTIONS

NOTES & RECIPE REVIEW

Serves	
Prep Time	
Cook Time	
Tools	
Temp	

Total	Carbs	Fat	Protein	Cals

KETO RECIPE

RECIPE NAME:

Keto	Low Carb	Paleo	Vegetarian	Vegan	Dairy Free	Gluten Free
☐	☐	☐	☐	☐	☐	☐

QTY	INGREDIENTS

RECIPE INSTRUCTIONS

NOTES & RECIPE REVIEW

Serves
Prep Time
Cook Time
Tools
Temp

Total	Carbs	Fat	Protein	Cals

KETO RECIPE

RECIPE NAME:

Keto	Low Carb	Paleo	Vegetarian	Vegan	Dairy Free	Gluten Free
☐	☐	☐	☐	☐	☐	☐

QTY	INGREDIENTS	RECIPE INSTRUCTIONS

NOTES & RECIPE REVIEW

Serves	
Prep Time	
Cook Time	
Tools	
Temp	

Total	Carbs	Fat	Protein	Cals

KETO RECIPE

RECIPE NAME:

Keto	Low Carb	Paleo	Vegetarian	Vegan	Dairy Free	Gluten Free
☐	☐	☐	☐	☐	☐	☐

QTY	INGREDIENTS	RECIPE INSTRUCTIONS

NOTES & RECIPE REVIEW

Serves	
Prep Time	
Cook Time	
Tools	
Temp	

Total	Carbs	Fat	Protein	Cals

KETO RECIPE

RECIPE NAME:

Keto	Low Carb	Paleo	Vegetarian	Vegan	Dairy Free	Gluten Free
☐	☐	☐	☐	☐	☐	☐

QTY	INGREDIENTS	RECIPE INSTRUCTIONS

NOTES & RECIPE REVIEW

Serves	
Prep Time	
Cook Time	
Tools	
Temp	

Total	Carbs	Fat	Protein	Cals

KETO RECIPE

RECIPE NAME:

Keto	Low Carb	Paleo	Vegetarian	Vegan	Dairy Free	Gluten Free
☐	☐	☐	☐	☐	☐	☐

QTY	INGREDIENTS	RECIPE INSTRUCTIONS

NOTES & RECIPE REVIEW

Serves	
Prep Time	
Cook Time	
Tools	
Temp	

Total	Carbs	Fat	Protein	Cals

KETO RECIPE

RECIPE NAME:

Keto	Low Carb	Paleo	Vegetarian	Vegan	Dairy Free	Gluten Free
☐	☐	☐	☐	☐	☐	☐

QTY	INGREDIENTS	RECIPE INSTRUCTIONS

NOTES & RECIPE REVIEW

Serves	
Prep Time	
Cook Time	
Tools	
Temp	

Total	Carbs	Fat	Protein	Cals

KETO RECIPE

RECIPE NAME:

Keto	Low Carb	Paleo	Vegetarian	Vegan	Dairy Free	Gluten Free
☐	☐	☐	☐	☐	☐	☐

QTY	INGREDIENTS	RECIPE INSTRUCTIONS

NOTES & RECIPE REVIEW

Serves	
Prep Time	
Cook Time	
Tools	
Temp	

Total	Carbs	Fat	Protein	Cals

KETO RECIPE

RECIPE NAME:

Keto	Low Carb	Paleo	Vegetarian	Vegan	Dairy Free	Gluten Free
☐	☐	☐	☐	☐	☐	☐

QTY	INGREDIENTS	RECIPE INSTRUCTIONS

NOTES & RECIPE REVIEW

Serves	
Prep Time	
Cook Time	
Tools	
Temp	

Total	Carbs	Fat	Protein	Cals

KETO RECIPE

RECIPE NAME:

Keto	Low Carb	Paleo	Vegetarian	Vegan	Dairy Free	Gluten Free
☐	☐	☐	☐	☐	☐	☐

QTY	INGREDIENTS	RECIPE INSTRUCTIONS

NOTES & RECIPE REVIEW

	Serves
	Prep Time
	Cook Time
	Tools
	Temp

Total	Carbs	Fat	Protein	Cals

KETO RECIPE

RECIPE NAME:

Keto	Low Carb	Paleo	Vegetarian	Vegan	Dairy Free	Gluten Free
☐	☐	☐	☐	☐	☐	☐

QTY	INGREDIENTS	RECIPE INSTRUCTIONS

NOTES & RECIPE REVIEW

Serves	
Prep Time	
Cook Time	
Tools	
Temp	

Total	Carbs	Fat	Protein	Cals

MACRO QUICK REFERENCE

MACRO TRACKER

QTY	TYPE	PROTEIN	FAT	CARBS	CALS	NOTES

MACRO QUICK REFERENCE

MACRO TRACKER

QTY	TYPE	PROTEIN	FAT	CARBS	CALS	NOTES

MACRO TRACKER

YEARLY KETO DAY TRACKER

JAN FEB MAR APR MAY JUN JUL AUG SEP OCT NOV DEC

1
2
3
4
5
6
7
8
9
10
11
12
13
14
15
16
17
18
19
20
21
22
23
24
25
26
27
28
29
30
31

COLOR IN THE DAYS THAT YOU WERE IN KETOSIS TO KEEP TRACK OF YOUR HEALTH AND WEIGHT LOSS PROGRESS!

NOTES & REFLECTIONS:

TOTAL DAYS IN KETOSIS:

MONTH ONE

IT'S ONLY 30 DAYS.
JUST DO IT FOR ONE DAY.
THEN DO IT FOR ONE DAY
AGAIN.

GOALS & ACCOMPLISHMENTS

MONTH JAN   FEB   MAR   APR   MAY   JUN   JUL   AUG   SEP   OCT   NOV   DEC

THIS MONTH'S GOALS

ACTION PLAN

M T W T F S S

WEEKLY GOALS

M
T
W
T
F
S
S

NOTES:

THOUGHTS

MEALS:	BREAKFAST	LUNCH	DINNER	SNACKS
M				
T				
W				
T				
F				
S				
S				

MONTHLY PROGRESS TRACKER

JAN FEB MAR APR MAY JUN JUL AUG SEP OCT NOV DEC

MON	TUE	WED	THU	FRI	SAT	SUN

WEIGHT LOSS MILESTONE TRACKER

CHEAT DAY TRACKER

WEEKLY DIET SUCCESS TRACKER & NOTES

WEEKLY FASTING TRACKER

Week Of: _______________

MONDAY

Goal	12	1	2	3	4	5	6	7	8	9	10	11	12	1	2	3	4	5	6	7	8	9	10	11
Actual	12	1	2	3	4	5	6	7	8	9	10	11	12	1	2	3	4	5	6	7	8	9	10	11

TUESDAY

Goal	12	1	2	3	4	5	6	7	8	9	10	11	12	1	2	3	4	5	6	7	8	9	10	11
Actual	12	1	2	3	4	5	6	7	8	9	10	11	12	1	2	3	4	5	6	7	8	9	10	11

WEDNESDAY

Goal	12	1	2	3	4	5	6	7	8	9	10	11	12	1	2	3	4	5	6	7	8	9	10	11
Actual	12	1	2	3	4	5	6	7	8	9	10	11	12	1	2	3	4	5	6	7	8	9	10	11

THURSDAY

Goal	12	1	2	3	4	5	6	7	8	9	10	11	12	1	2	3	4	5	6	7	8	9	10	11
Actual	12	1	2	3	4	5	6	7	8	9	10	11	12	1	2	3	4	5	6	7	8	9	10	11

FRIDAY

Goal	12	1	2	3	4	5	6	7	8	9	10	11	12	1	2	3	4	5	6	7	8	9	10	11
Actual	12	1	2	3	4	5	6	7	8	9	10	11	12	1	2	3	4	5	6	7	8	9	10	11

SATURDAY

Goal	12	1	2	3	4	5	6	7	8	9	10	11	12	1	2	3	4	5	6	7	8	9	10	11
Actual	12	1	2	3	4	5	6	7	8	9	10	11	12	1	2	3	4	5	6	7	8	9	10	11

SUNDAY

Goal	12	1	2	3	4	5	6	7	8	9	10	11	12	1	2	3	4	5	6	7	8	9	10	11
Actual	12	1	2	3	4	5	6	7	8	9	10	11	12	1	2	3	4	5	6	7	8	9	10	11

WEEKLY MEAL PLANNER

Week of: ___________

	Breakfast	Lunch	Dinner	Snack	Other
Monday	TOTAL Carbs Fat Protein Cals	TOTAL Carbs Fat Protein Cals	TOTAL Carbs Fat Protein Cals	TOTAL Carbs Fat Protein Cals	TOTAL Carbs Fat Protein Cals
Tuesday	TOTAL Carbs Fat Protein Cals	TOTAL Carbs Fat Protein Cals	TOTAL Carbs Fat Protein Cals	TOTAL Carbs Fat Protein Cals	TOTAL Carbs Fat Protein Cals
Wednesday	TOTAL Carbs Fat Protein Cals	TOTAL Carbs Fat Protein Cals	TOTAL Carbs Fat Protein Cals	TOTAL Carbs Fat Protein Cals	TOTAL Carbs Fat Protein Cals
Thursday	TOTAL Carbs Fat Protein Cals	TOTAL Carbs Fat Protein Cals	TOTAL Carbs Fat Protein Cals	TOTAL Carbs Fat Protein Cals	TOTAL Carbs Fat Protein Cals
Friday	TOTAL Carbs Fat Protein Cals	TOTAL Carbs Fat Protein Cals	TOTAL Carbs Fat Protein Cals	TOTAL Carbs Fat Protein Cals	TOTAL Carbs Fat Protein Cals
Saturday	TOTAL Carbs Fat Protein Cals	TOTAL Carbs Fat Protein Cals	TOTAL Carbs Fat Protein Cals	TOTAL Carbs Fat Protein Cals	TOTAL Carbs Fat Protein Cals
Sunday	TOTAL Carbs Fat Protein Cals	TOTAL Carbs Fat Protein Cals	TOTAL Carbs Fat Protein Cals	TOTAL Carbs Fat Protein Cals	TOTAL Carbs Fat Protein Cals

WEEKLY LOW CARB SHOPPING LIST

FRESH PRODUCE

MEAT AND SEAFOOD

DAIRY PRODUCTS

PANTRY ITEMS

FROZEN / OTHER

DAILY PROGRESS TRACKER

SLEEP TRACKER:

DATE

RISE:

BEDTIME:

SLEEP (HRS):

NOTES FOR THE DAY

IN A STATE OF KETOSIS?

YES   NO   UNSURE

WATER INTAKE TRACKER

EXERCISE / WORKOUT ROUTINE

DAILY ENERGY LEVEL

HIGH   MEDIUM   LOW

BREAKFAST

FAT: CARBS: PROTEIN: CALORIES:

LUNCH

FAT: CARBS: PROTEIN: CALORIES:

DINNER

FAT: CARBS: PROTEIN: CALORIES:

SNACKS

FAT: CARBS: PROTEIN: CALORIES:

HOW DO I FEEL TODAY?

TOP 6 PRIORITIES OF THE DAY

END OF THE DAY TOTAL OVERVIEW

CARBS   FAT   PROTEIN   CALORIES

DAILY PROGRESS TRACKER

SLEEP TRACKER:

DATE _______________

RISE: ________   BEDTIME: ________   SLEEP (HRS): ________

NOTES FOR THE DAY

IN A STATE OF KETOSIS?

YES   NO   UNSURE

WATER INTAKE TRACKER

EXERCISE / WORKOUT ROUTINE

DAILY ENERGY LEVEL

HIGH   MEDIUM   LOW

BREAKFAST

FAT: CARBS: PROTEIN: CALORIES:

LUNCH

FAT: CARBS: PROTEIN: CALORIES:

DINNER

FAT: CARBS: PROTEIN: CALORIES:

HOW DO I FEEL TODAY?

SNACKS

FAT: CARBS: PROTEIN: CALORIES:

TOP 6 PRIORITIES OF THE DAY

END OF THE DAY TOTAL OVERVIEW

CARBS   FAT   PROTEIN   CALORIES

DAILY PROGRESS TRACKER

SLEEP TRACKER:

DATE _______________

RISE: BEDTIME: SLEEP (HRS):

NOTES FOR THE DAY

IN A STATE OF KETOSIS?

YES   NO   UNSURE

WATER INTAKE TRACKER

EXERCISE / WORKOUT ROUTINE

DAILY ENERGY LEVEL

HIGH   **MEDIUM**   **LOW**

BREAKFAST

FAT: CARBS: PROTEIN: CALORIES:

LUNCH

FAT: CARBS: PROTEIN: CALORIES:

DINNER

FAT: CARBS: PROTEIN: CALORIES:

SNACKS

FAT: CARBS: PROTEIN: CALORIES:

HOW DO I FEEL TODAY?

TOP 6 PRIORITIES OF THE DAY

END OF THE DAY TOTAL OVERVIEW

CARBS   FAT   PROTEIN   CALORIES

DAILY PROGRESS TRACKER

SLEEP TRACKER:

DATE

RISE:

BEDTIME:

SLEEP (HRS):

NOTES FOR THE DAY

IN A STATE OF KETOSIS?

YES   NO   UNSURE

WATER INTAKE TRACKER

EXERCISE / WORKOUT ROUTINE

DAILY ENERGY LEVEL

HIGH   **MEDIUM**   **LOW**

BREAKFAST

FAT: CARBS: PROTEIN: CALORIES:

LUNCH

FAT: CARBS: PROTEIN: CALORIES:

HOW DO I FEEL TODAY?

DINNER

FAT: CARBS: PROTEIN: CALORIES:

SNACKS

FAT: CARBS: PROTEIN: CALORIES:

TOP 6 PRIORITIES OF THE DAY

END OF THE DAY TOTAL OVERVIEW

CARBS   FAT   PROTEIN   CALORIES

DAILY PROGRESS TRACKER

SLEEP TRACKER:

DATE

RISE:

BEDTIME:

SLEEP (HRS):

NOTES FOR THE DAY

IN A STATE OF KETOSIS?

YES   NO   UNSURE

WATER INTAKE TRACKER

EXERCISE / WORKOUT ROUTINE

DAILY ENERGY LEVEL

HIGH   **MEDIUM**   **LOW**

BREAKFAST

FAT: CARBS: PROTEIN: CALORIES:

LUNCH

FAT: CARBS: PROTEIN: CALORIES:

HOW DO I FEEL TODAY?

DINNER

FAT: CARBS: PROTEIN: CALORIES:

SNACKS

FAT: CARBS: PROTEIN: CALORIES:

TOP 6 PRIORITIES OF THE DAY

END OF THE DAY TOTAL OVERVIEW

CARBS   FAT   PROTEIN   CALORIES

DAILY PROGRESS TRACKER

SLEEP TRACKER:

DATE ___________

RISE: ___________ BEDTIME: ___________ SLEEP (HRS): ___________

NOTES FOR THE DAY

IN A STATE OF KETOSIS?

YES   NO   UNSURE

WATER INTAKE TRACKER

EXERCISE / WORKOUT ROUTINE

DAILY ENERGY LEVEL

HIGH   **MEDIUM**   **LOW**

BREAKFAST

FAT: CARBS: PROTEIN: CALORIES:

LUNCH

FAT: CARBS: PROTEIN: CALORIES:

DINNER

FAT: CARBS: PROTEIN: CALORIES:

SNACKS

FAT: CARBS: PROTEIN: CALORIES:

HOW DO I FEEL TODAY?

TOP 6 PRIORITIES OF THE DAY

END OF THE DAY TOTAL OVERVIEW

CARBS   FAT   PROTEIN   CALORIES

DAILY PROGRESS TRACKER

SLEEP TRACKER:

DATE

RISE: BEDTIME: SLEEP (HRS):

NOTES FOR THE DAY

EXERCISE / WORKOUT ROUTINE

HOW DO I FEEL TODAY?

TOP 6 PRIORITIES OF THE DAY

IN A STATE OF KETOSIS?

YES   NO   UNSURE

WATER INTAKE TRACKER

DAILY ENERGY LEVEL

HIGH   MEDIUM   LOW

BREAKFAST

FAT: CARBS: PROTEIN: CALORIES:

LUNCH

FAT: CARBS: PROTEIN: CALORIES:

DINNER

FAT: CARBS: PROTEIN: CALORIES:

SNACKS

FAT: CARBS: PROTEIN: CALORIES:

END OF THE DAY TOTAL OVERVIEW

CARBS   FAT   PROTEIN   CALORIES

WEEKLY FASTING TRACKER

Week Of: _______________

MONDAY

Goal	12	1	2	3	4	5	6	7	8	9	10	11	12	1	2	3	4	5	6	7	8	9	10	11
Actual	12	1	2	3	4	5	6	7	8	9	10	11	12	1	2	3	4	5	6	7	8	9	10	11

TUESDAY

Goal	12	1	2	3	4	5	6	7	8	9	10	11	12	1	2	3	4	5	6	7	8	9	10	11
Actual	12	1	2	3	4	5	6	7	8	9	10	11	12	1	2	3	4	5	6	7	8	9	10	11

WEDNESDAY

Goal	12	1	2	3	4	5	6	7	8	9	10	11	12	1	2	3	4	5	6	7	8	9	10	11
Actual	12	1	2	3	4	5	6	7	8	9	10	11	12	1	2	3	4	5	6	7	8	9	10	11

THURSDAY

Goal	12	1	2	3	4	5	6	7	8	9	10	11	12	1	2	3	4	5	6	7	8	9	10	11
Actual	12	1	2	3	4	5	6	7	8	9	10	11	12	1	2	3	4	5	6	7	8	9	10	11

FRIDAY

Goal	12	1	2	3	4	5	6	7	8	9	10	11	12	1	2	3	4	5	6	7	8	9	10	11
Actual	12	1	2	3	4	5	6	7	8	9	10	11	12	1	2	3	4	5	6	7	8	9	10	11

SATURDAY

Goal	12	1	2	3	4	5	6	7	8	9	10	11	12	1	2	3	4	5	6	7	8	9	10	11
Actual	12	1	2	3	4	5	6	7	8	9	10	11	12	1	2	3	4	5	6	7	8	9	10	11

SUNDAY

Goal	12	1	2	3	4	5	6	7	8	9	10	11	12	1	2	3	4	5	6	7	8	9	10	11
Actual	12	1	2	3	4	5	6	7	8	9	10	11	12	1	2	3	4	5	6	7	8	9	10	11

WEEKLY MEAL PLANNER

Week of: _______________

	Breakfast	Lunch	Dinner	Snack	Other
Monday	TOTAL Carbs Fat Protein Cals	TOTAL Carbs Fat Protein Cals	TOTAL Carbs Fat Protein Cals	TOTAL Carbs Fat Protein Cals	TOTAL Carbs Fat Protein Cals
Tuesday	TOTAL Carbs Fat Protein Cals	TOTAL Carbs Fat Protein Cals	TOTAL Carbs Fat Protein Cals	TOTAL Carbs Fat Protein Cals	TOTAL Carbs Fat Protein Cals
Wednesday	TOTAL Carbs Fat Protein Cals	TOTAL Carbs Fat Protein Cals	TOTAL Carbs Fat Protein Cals	TOTAL Carbs Fat Protein Cals	TOTAL Carbs Fat Protein Cals
Thursday	TOTAL Carbs Fat Protein Cals	TOTAL Carbs Fat Protein Cals	TOTAL Carbs Fat Protein Cals	TOTAL Carbs Fat Protein Cals	TOTAL Carbs Fat Protein Cals
Friday	TOTAL Carbs Fat Protein Cals	TOTAL Carbs Fat Protein Cals	TOTAL Carbs Fat Protein Cals	TOTAL Carbs Fat Protein Cals	TOTAL Carbs Fat Protein Cals
Saturday	TOTAL Carbs Fat Protein Cals	TOTAL Carbs Fat Protein Cals	TOTAL Carbs Fat Protein Cals	TOTAL Carbs Fat Protein Cals	TOTAL Carbs Fat Protein Cals
Sunday	TOTAL Carbs Fat Protein Cals	TOTAL Carbs Fat Protein Cals	TOTAL Carbs Fat Protein Cals	TOTAL Carbs Fat Protein Cals	TOTAL Carbs Fat Protein Cals

WEEKLY LOW CARB SHOPPING LIST

FRESH PRODUCE

MEAT AND SEAFOOD

DAIRY PRODUCTS

PANTRY ITEMS

FROZEN / OTHER

DAILY PROGRESS TRACKER

SLEEP TRACKER:

DATE

RISE: BEDTIME: SLEEP (HRS):

NOTES FOR THE DAY

IN A STATE OF KETOSIS?

YES   NO   UNSURE

WATER INTAKE TRACKER

EXERCISE / WORKOUT ROUTINE

DAILY ENERGY LEVEL

HIGH   **MEDIUM**   **LOW**

BREAKFAST

FAT: CARBS: PROTEIN: CALORIES:

LUNCH

FAT: CARBS: PROTEIN: CALORIES:

DINNER

FAT: CARBS: PROTEIN: CALORIES:

SNACKS

FAT: CARBS: PROTEIN: CALORIES:

HOW DO I FEEL TODAY?

TOP 6 PRIORITIES OF THE DAY

END OF THE DAY TOTAL OVERVIEW

CARBS   FAT   PROTEIN   CALORIES

DAILY PROGRESS TRACKER

SLEEP TRACKER:

DATE ______________

RISE: BEDTIME: SLEEP (HRS):

NOTES FOR THE DAY

EXERCISE / WORKOUT ROUTINE

HOW DO I FEEL TODAY?

TOP 6 PRIORITIES OF THE DAY

IN A STATE OF KETOSIS?

YES   NO   UNSURE

WATER INTAKE TRACKER

DAILY ENERGY LEVEL

HIGH   **MEDIUM**   **LOW**

BREAKFAST

FAT: CARBS: PROTEIN: CALORIES:

LUNCH

FAT: CARBS: PROTEIN: CALORIES:

DINNER

FAT: CARBS: PROTEIN: CALORIES:

SNACKS

FAT: CARBS: PROTEIN: CALORIES:

END OF THE DAY TOTAL OVERVIEW

CARBS   FAT   PROTEIN   CALORIES

DAILY PROGRESS TRACKER

SLEEP TRACKER:

DATE ___________

RISE: _______ BEDTIME: _______ SLEEP (HRS): _______

NOTES FOR THE DAY

IN A STATE OF KETOSIS?

YES   NO   UNSURE

WATER INTAKE TRACKER

EXERCISE / WORKOUT ROUTINE

DAILY ENERGY LEVEL		
HIGH	MEDIUM	LOW

BREAKFAST

FAT: CARBS: PROTEIN: CALORIES:

LUNCH

FAT: CARBS: PROTEIN: CALORIES:

HOW DO I FEEL TODAY?

DINNER

FAT: CARBS: PROTEIN: CALORIES:

SNACKS

FAT: CARBS: PROTEIN: CALORIES:

TOP 6 PRIORITIES OF THE DAY

END OF THE DAY TOTAL OVERVIEW

CARBS   FAT   PROTEIN   CALORIES

DAILY PROGRESS TRACKER

SLEEP TRACKER:

DATE ________

RISE: | BEDTIME: | SLEEP (HRS):

NOTES FOR THE DAY

IN A STATE OF KETOSIS?

YES   NO   UNSURE

WATER INTAKE TRACKER

EXERCISE / WORKOUT ROUTINE

DAILY ENERGY LEVEL		
HIGH	**MEDIUM**	**LOW**

BREAKFAST

FAT: CARBS: PROTEIN: CALORIES:

LUNCH

FAT: CARBS: PROTEIN: CALORIES:

HOW DO I FEEL TODAY?

DINNER

FAT: CARBS: PROTEIN: CALORIES:

SNACKS

FAT: CARBS: PROTEIN: CALORIES:

TOP 6 PRIORITIES OF THE DAY

END OF THE DAY TOTAL OVERVIEW

CARBS   FAT   PROTEIN   CALORIES

DAILY PROGRESS TRACKER

SLEEP TRACKER:

DATE _______________

RISE: ________   BEDTIME: ________   SLEEP (HRS): ________

NOTES FOR THE DAY

IN A STATE OF KETOSIS?

YES   NO   UNSURE

WATER INTAKE TRACKER

EXERCISE / WORKOUT ROUTINE

DAILY ENERGY LEVEL		
HIGH	MEDIUM	LOW

BREAKFAST

FAT: CARBS: PROTEIN: CALORIES:

LUNCH

FAT: CARBS: PROTEIN: CALORIES:

DINNER

FAT: CARBS: PROTEIN: CALORIES:

SNACKS

FAT: CARBS: PROTEIN: CALORIES:

HOW DO I FEEL TODAY?

TOP 6 PRIORITIES OF THE DAY

END OF THE DAY TOTAL OVERVIEW

CARBS   FAT   PROTEIN   CALORIES

DAILY PROGRESS TRACKER

SLEEP TRACKER:

RISE: | BEDTIME: | SLEEP (HRS):

DATE

NOTES FOR THE DAY

EXERCISE / WORKOUT ROUTINE

HOW DO I FEEL TODAY?

TOP 6 PRIORITIES OF THE DAY

IN A STATE OF KETOSIS?

YES   NO   UNSURE

WATER INTAKE TRACKER

DAILY ENERGY LEVEL

HIGH   MEDIUM   LOW

BREAKFAST

FAT: CARBS: PROTEIN: CALORIES:

LUNCH

FAT: CARBS: PROTEIN: CALORIES:

DINNER

FAT: CARBS: PROTEIN: CALORIES:

SNACKS

FAT: CARBS: PROTEIN: CALORIES:

END OF THE DAY TOTAL OVERVIEW

CARBS   FAT   PROTEIN   CALORIES

DAILY PROGRESS TRACKER

SLEEP TRACKER:

DATE ________________

RISE: __________   BEDTIME: __________   SLEEP (HRS): __________

NOTES FOR THE DAY

____

____

____

EXERCISE / WORKOUT ROUTINE

HOW DO I FEEL TODAY?

TOP 6 PRIORITIES OF THE DAY

IN A STATE OF KETOSIS?

YES   NO   UNSURE

WATER INTAKE TRACKER

DAILY ENERGY LEVEL		
HIGH	MEDIUM	LOW

BREAKFAST

FAT: CARBS: PROTEIN: CALORIES:

LUNCH

FAT: CARBS: PROTEIN: CALORIES:

DINNER

FAT: CARBS: PROTEIN: CALORIES:

SNACKS

FAT: CARBS: PROTEIN: CALORIES:

END OF THE DAY TOTAL OVERVIEW

CARBS   FAT   PROTEIN   CALORIES

WEEKLY FASTING TRACKER

Week Of: ___________________

MONDAY

| Goal | 12 | 1 | 2 | 3 | 4 | 5 | 6 | 7 | 8 | 9 | 10 | 11 | 12 | 1 | 2 | 3 | 4 | 5 | 6 | 7 | 8 | 9 | 10 | 11 |
| Actual | 12 | 1 | 2 | 3 | 4 | 5 | 6 | 7 | 8 | 9 | 10 | 11 | 12 | 1 | 2 | 3 | 4 | 5 | 6 | 7 | 8 | 9 | 10 | 11 |

TUESDAY

| Goal | 12 | 1 | 2 | 3 | 4 | 5 | 6 | 7 | 8 | 9 | 10 | 11 | 12 | 1 | 2 | 3 | 4 | 5 | 6 | 7 | 8 | 9 | 10 | 11 |
| Actual | 12 | 1 | 2 | 3 | 4 | 5 | 6 | 7 | 8 | 9 | 10 | 11 | 12 | 1 | 2 | 3 | 4 | 5 | 6 | 7 | 8 | 9 | 10 | 11 |

WEDNESDAY

| Goal | 12 | 1 | 2 | 3 | 4 | 5 | 6 | 7 | 8 | 9 | 10 | 11 | 12 | 1 | 2 | 3 | 4 | 5 | 6 | 7 | 8 | 9 | 10 | 11 |
| Actual | 12 | 1 | 2 | 3 | 4 | 5 | 6 | 7 | 8 | 9 | 10 | 11 | 12 | 1 | 2 | 3 | 4 | 5 | 6 | 7 | 8 | 9 | 10 | 11 |

THURSDAY

| Goal | 12 | 1 | 2 | 3 | 4 | 5 | 6 | 7 | 8 | 9 | 10 | 11 | 12 | 1 | 2 | 3 | 4 | 5 | 6 | 7 | 8 | 9 | 10 | 11 |
| Actual | 12 | 1 | 2 | 3 | 4 | 5 | 6 | 7 | 8 | 9 | 10 | 11 | 12 | 1 | 2 | 3 | 4 | 5 | 6 | 7 | 8 | 9 | 10 | 11 |

FRIDAY

| Goal | 12 | 1 | 2 | 3 | 4 | 5 | 6 | 7 | 8 | 9 | 10 | 11 | 12 | 1 | 2 | 3 | 4 | 5 | 6 | 7 | 8 | 9 | 10 | 11 |
| Actual | 12 | 1 | 2 | 3 | 4 | 5 | 6 | 7 | 8 | 9 | 10 | 11 | 12 | 1 | 2 | 3 | 4 | 5 | 6 | 7 | 8 | 9 | 10 | 11 |

SATURDAY

| Goal | 12 | 1 | 2 | 3 | 4 | 5 | 6 | 7 | 8 | 9 | 10 | 11 | 12 | 1 | 2 | 3 | 4 | 5 | 6 | 7 | 8 | 9 | 10 | 11 |
| Actual | 12 | 1 | 2 | 3 | 4 | 5 | 6 | 7 | 8 | 9 | 10 | 11 | 12 | 1 | 2 | 3 | 4 | 5 | 6 | 7 | 8 | 9 | 10 | 11 |

SUNDAY

| Goal | 12 | 1 | 2 | 3 | 4 | 5 | 6 | 7 | 8 | 9 | 10 | 11 | 12 | 1 | 2 | 3 | 4 | 5 | 6 | 7 | 8 | 9 | 10 | 11 |
| Actual | 12 | 1 | 2 | 3 | 4 | 5 | 6 | 7 | 8 | 9 | 10 | 11 | 12 | 1 | 2 | 3 | 4 | 5 | 6 | 7 | 8 | 9 | 10 | 11 |

WEEKLY MEAL PLANNER

Week of: _______________

	Breakfast	Lunch	Dinner	Snack	Other
Monday	TOTAL Carbs Fat Protein Cals	TOTAL Carbs Fat Protein Cals	TOTAL Carbs Fat Protein Cals	TOTAL Carbs Fat Protein Cals	TOTAL Carbs Fat Protein Cals
Tuesday	TOTAL Carbs Fat Protein Cals	TOTAL Carbs Fat Protein Cals	TOTAL Carbs Fat Protein Cals	TOTAL Carbs Fat Protein Cals	TOTAL Carbs Fat Protein Cals
Wednesday	TOTAL Carbs Fat Protein Cals	TOTAL Carbs Fat Protein Cals	TOTAL Carbs Fat Protein Cals	TOTAL Carbs Fat Protein Cals	TOTAL Carbs Fat Protein Cals
Thursday	TOTAL Carbs Fat Protein Cals	TOTAL Carbs Fat Protein Cals	TOTAL Carbs Fat Protein Cals	TOTAL Carbs Fat Protein Cals	TOTAL Carbs Fat Protein Cals
Friday	TOTAL Carbs Fat Protein Cals	TOTAL Carbs Fat Protein Cals	TOTAL Carbs Fat Protein Cals	TOTAL Carbs Fat Protein Cals	TOTAL Carbs Fat Protein Cals
Saturday	TOTAL Carbs Fat Protein Cals	TOTAL Carbs Fat Protein Cals	TOTAL Carbs Fat Protein Cals	TOTAL Carbs Fat Protein Cals	TOTAL Carbs Fat Protein Cals
Sunday	TOTAL Carbs Fat Protein Cals	TOTAL Carbs Fat Protein Cals	TOTAL Carbs Fat Protein Cals	TOTAL Carbs Fat Protein Cals	TOTAL Carbs Fat Protein Cals

WEEKLY LOW CARB SHOPPING LIST

FRESH PRODUCE

MEAT AND SEAFOOD

DAIRY PRODUCTS

PANTRY ITEMS

FROZEN / OTHER

DAILY PROGRESS TRACKER

SLEEP TRACKER:

DATE

RISE:　　　BEDTIME:　　　SLEEP (HRS):

NOTES FOR THE DAY

IN A STATE OF KETOSIS?

YES　　　NO　　　UNSURE

WATER INTAKE TRACKER

EXERCISE / WORKOUT ROUTINE

DAILY ENERGY LEVEL

HIGH　　　MEDIUM　　　LOW

BREAKFAST

FAT:　　CARBS:　　PROTEIN:　　CALORIES:

LUNCH

FAT:　　CARBS:　　PROTEIN:　　CALORIES:

DINNER

FAT:　　CARBS:　　PROTEIN:　　CALORIES:

SNACKS

FAT:　　CARBS:　　PROTEIN:　　CALORIES:

HOW DO I FEEL TODAY?

TOP 6 PRIORITIES OF THE DAY

END OF THE DAY TOTAL OVERVIEW

CARBS　　　FAT　　　PROTEIN　　　CALORIES

DAILY PROGRESS TRACKER

SLEEP TRACKER:

DATE

RISE:

BEDTIME:

SLEEP (HRS):

NOTES FOR THE DAY

IN A STATE OF KETOSIS?

YES   NO   UNSURE

WATER INTAKE TRACKER

EXERCISE / WORKOUT ROUTINE

DAILY ENERGY LEVEL

HIGH   **MEDIUM**   **LOW**

BREAKFAST

FAT: CARBS: PROTEIN: CALORIES:

LUNCH

FAT: CARBS: PROTEIN: CALORIES:

HOW DO I FEEL TODAY?

DINNER

FAT: CARBS: PROTEIN: CALORIES:

SNACKS

FAT: CARBS: PROTEIN: CALORIES:

TOP 6 PRIORITIES OF THE DAY

END OF THE DAY TOTAL OVERVIEW

CARBS   FAT   PROTEIN   CALORIES

DAILY PROGRESS TRACKER

SLEEP TRACKER:

RISE:

BEDTIME:

DATE

SLEEP (HRS):

NOTES FOR THE DAY

IN A STATE OF KETOSIS?

YES   NO   UNSURE

WATER INTAKE TRACKER

EXERCISE / WORKOUT ROUTINE

DAILY ENERGY LEVEL		
HIGH	MEDIUM	LOW

BREAKFAST

FAT: CARBS: PROTEIN: CALORIES:

LUNCH

FAT: CARBS: PROTEIN: CALORIES:

HOW DO I FEEL TODAY?

DINNER

FAT: CARBS: PROTEIN: CALORIES:

SNACKS

FAT: CARBS: PROTEIN: CALORIES:

TOP 6 PRIORITIES OF THE DAY

END OF THE DAY TOTAL OVERVIEW

CARBS   FAT   PROTEIN   CALORIES

DAILY PROGRESS TRACKER

SLEEP TRACKER:

RISE: BEDTIME: SLEEP (HRS):

DATE

NOTES FOR THE DAY

EXERCISE / WORKOUT ROUTINE

HOW DO I FEEL TODAY?

TOP 6 PRIORITIES OF THE DAY

IN A STATE OF KETOSIS?

YES   NO   UNSURE

WATER INTAKE TRACKER

DAILY ENERGY LEVEL

HIGH   MEDIUM   LOW

BREAKFAST

FAT: CARBS: PROTEIN: CALORIES:

LUNCH

FAT: CARBS: PROTEIN: CALORIES:

DINNER

FAT: CARBS: PROTEIN: CALORIES:

SNACKS

FAT: CARBS: PROTEIN: CALORIES:

END OF THE DAY TOTAL OVERVIEW

CARBS   FAT   PROTEIN   CALORIES

DAILY PROGRESS TRACKER

SLEEP TRACKER:

DATE

RISE:

BEDTIME:

SLEEP (HRS):

NOTES FOR THE DAY

IN A STATE OF KETOSIS?

YES   NO   UNSURE

WATER INTAKE TRACKER

EXERCISE / WORKOUT ROUTINE

DAILY ENERGY LEVEL		
HIGH	**MEDIUM**	**LOW**

BREAKFAST

FAT: CARBS: PROTEIN: CALORIES:

LUNCH

FAT: CARBS: PROTEIN: CALORIES:

DINNER

FAT: CARBS: PROTEIN: CALORIES:

SNACKS

FAT: CARBS: PROTEIN: CALORIES:

HOW DO I FEEL TODAY?

TOP 6 PRIORITIES OF THE DAY

END OF THE DAY TOTAL OVERVIEW

CARBS   FAT   PROTEIN   CALORIES

DAILY PROGRESS TRACKER

SLEEP TRACKER:

DATE

RISE:

BEDTIME:

SLEEP (HRS):

NOTES FOR THE DAY

IN A STATE OF KETOSIS?

YES   NO   UNSURE

WATER INTAKE TRACKER

EXERCISE / WORKOUT ROUTINE

DAILY ENERGY LEVEL

HIGH   **MEDIUM**   **LOW**

BREAKFAST

FAT: CARBS: PROTEIN: CALORIES:

LUNCH

FAT: CARBS: PROTEIN: CALORIES:

HOW DO I FEEL TODAY?

DINNER

FAT: CARBS: PROTEIN: CALORIES:

SNACKS

FAT: CARBS: PROTEIN: CALORIES:

TOP 6 PRIORITIES OF THE DAY

END OF THE DAY TOTAL OVERVIEW

CARBS   FAT   PROTEIN   CALORIES

DAILY PROGRESS TRACKER

SLEEP TRACKER:

DATE ___________

RISE: | BEDTIME: | SLEEP (HRS):

NOTES FOR THE DAY

IN A STATE OF KETOSIS?

YES   NO   UNSURE

WATER INTAKE TRACKER

EXERCISE / WORKOUT ROUTINE

DAILY ENERGY LEVEL

HIGH   **MEDIUM**   **LOW**

BREAKFAST

FAT: CARBS: PROTEIN: CALORIES:

LUNCH

FAT: CARBS: PROTEIN: CALORIES:

DINNER

FAT: CARBS: PROTEIN: CALORIES:

SNACKS

FAT: CARBS: PROTEIN: CALORIES:

HOW DO I FEEL TODAY?

TOP 6 PRIORITIES OF THE DAY

END OF THE DAY TOTAL OVERVIEW

CARBS   FAT   PROTEIN   CALORIES

WEEKLY FASTING TRACKER

Week Of: _______________________

MONDAY

Goal	12	1	2	3	4	5	6	7	8	9	10	11	12	1	2	3	4	5	6	7	8	9	10	11
Actual	12	1	2	3	4	5	6	7	8	9	10	11	12	1	2	3	4	5	6	7	8	9	10	11

TUESDAY

Goal	12	1	2	3	4	5	6	7	8	9	10	11	12	1	2	3	4	5	6	7	8	9	10	11
Actual	12	1	2	3	4	5	6	7	8	9	10	11	12	1	2	3	4	5	6	7	8	9	10	11

WEDNESDAY

Goal	12	1	2	3	4	5	6	7	8	9	10	11	12	1	2	3	4	5	6	7	8	9	10	11
Actual	12	1	2	3	4	5	6	7	8	9	10	11	12	1	2	3	4	5	6	7	8	9	10	11

THURSDAY

Goal	12	1	2	3	4	5	6	7	8	9	10	11	12	1	2	3	4	5	6	7	8	9	10	11
Actual	12	1	2	3	4	5	6	7	8	9	10	11	12	1	2	3	4	5	6	7	8	9	10	11

FRIDAY

Goal	12	1	2	3	4	5	6	7	8	9	10	11	12	1	2	3	4	5	6	7	8	9	10	11
Actual	12	1	2	3	4	5	6	7	8	9	10	11	12	1	2	3	4	5	6	7	8	9	10	11

SATURDAY

Goal	12	1	2	3	4	5	6	7	8	9	10	11	12	1	2	3	4	5	6	7	8	9	10	11
Actual	12	1	2	3	4	5	6	7	8	9	10	11	12	1	2	3	4	5	6	7	8	9	10	11

SUNDAY

Goal	12	1	2	3	4	5	6	7	8	9	10	11	12	1	2	3	4	5	6	7	8	9	10	11
Actual	12	1	2	3	4	5	6	7	8	9	10	11	12	1	2	3	4	5	6	7	8	9	10	11

WEEKLY MEAL PLANNER

Week of: _______________

	Breakfast	Lunch	Dinner	Snack	Other
Monday	TOTAL Carbs Fat Protein Cals	TOTAL Carbs Fat Protein Cals	TOTAL Carbs Fat Protein Cals	TOTAL Carbs Fat Protein Cals	TOTAL Carbs Fat Protein Cals
Tuesday	TOTAL Carbs Fat Protein Cals	TOTAL Carbs Fat Protein Cals	TOTAL Carbs Fat Protein Cals	TOTAL Carbs Fat Protein Cals	TOTAL Carbs Fat Protein Cals
Wednesday	TOTAL Carbs Fat Protein Cals	TOTAL Carbs Fat Protein Cals	TOTAL Carbs Fat Protein Cals	TOTAL Carbs Fat Protein Cals	TOTAL Carbs Fat Protein Cals
Thursday	TOTAL Carbs Fat Protein Cals	TOTAL Carbs Fat Protein Cals	TOTAL Carbs Fat Protein Cals	TOTAL Carbs Fat Protein Cals	TOTAL Carbs Fat Protein Cals
Friday	TOTAL Carbs Fat Protein Cals	TOTAL Carbs Fat Protein Cals	TOTAL Carbs Fat Protein Cals	TOTAL Carbs Fat Protein Cals	TOTAL Carbs Fat Protein Cals
Saturday	TOTAL Carbs Fat Protein Cals	TOTAL Carbs Fat Protein Cals	TOTAL Carbs Fat Protein Cals	TOTAL Carbs Fat Protein Cals	TOTAL Carbs Fat Protein Cals
Sunday	TOTAL Carbs Fat Protein Cals	TOTAL Carbs Fat Protein Cals	TOTAL Carbs Fat Protein Cals	TOTAL Carbs Fat Protein Cals	TOTAL Carbs Fat Protein Cals

WEEKLY LOW CARB SHOPPING LIST

FRESH PRODUCE

MEAT AND SEAFOOD

DAIRY PRODUCTS

PANTRY ITEMS

FROZEN / OTHER

DAILY PROGRESS TRACKER

SLEEP TRACKER:

DATE

RISE:

BEDTIME:

SLEEP (HRS):

NOTES FOR THE DAY

IN A STATE OF KETOSIS?

YES   NO   UNSURE

WATER INTAKE TRACKER

EXERCISE / WORKOUT ROUTINE

DAILY ENERGY LEVEL

HIGH   MEDIUM   LOW

BREAKFAST

FAT: CARBS: PROTEIN: CALORIES:

LUNCH

FAT: CARBS: PROTEIN: CALORIES:

HOW DO I FEEL TODAY?

DINNER

FAT: CARBS: PROTEIN: CALORIES:

SNACKS

FAT: CARBS: PROTEIN: CALORIES:

TOP 6 PRIORITIES OF THE DAY

END OF THE DAY TOTAL OVERVIEW

CARBS   FAT   PROTEIN   CALORIES

DAILY PROGRESS TRACKER

SLEEP TRACKER:

DATE ___________

RISE: _______   BEDTIME: _______   SLEEP (HRS): _______

NOTES FOR THE DAY

IN A STATE OF KETOSIS?

YES   NO   UNSURE

WATER INTAKE TRACKER

EXERCISE / WORKOUT ROUTINE

DAILY ENERGY LEVEL		
HIGH	**MEDIUM**	**LOW**

BREAKFAST

FAT: CARBS: PROTEIN: CALORIES:

LUNCH

FAT: CARBS: PROTEIN: CALORIES:

HOW DO I FEEL TODAY?

DINNER

FAT: CARBS: PROTEIN: CALORIES:

SNACKS

FAT: CARBS: PROTEIN: CALORIES:

TOP 6 PRIORITIES OF THE DAY

END OF THE DAY TOTAL OVERVIEW

CARBS   FAT   PROTEIN   CALORIES

DAILY PROGRESS TRACKER

SLEEP TRACKER:

DATE

RISE:

BEDTIME:

SLEEP (HRS):

NOTES FOR THE DAY

IN A STATE OF KETOSIS?

YES   NO   UNSURE

WATER INTAKE TRACKER

EXERCISE / WORKOUT ROUTINE

DAILY ENERGY LEVEL

HIGH   **MEDIUM**   **LOW**

BREAKFAST

FAT: CARBS: PROTEIN: CALORIES:

LUNCH

FAT: CARBS: PROTEIN: CALORIES:

DINNER

FAT: CARBS: PROTEIN: CALORIES:

SNACKS

FAT: CARBS: PROTEIN: CALORIES:

HOW DO I FEEL TODAY?

TOP 6 PRIORITIES OF THE DAY

END OF THE DAY TOTAL OVERVIEW

CARBS   FAT   PROTEIN   CALORIES

DAILY PROGRESS TRACKER

SLEEP TRACKER:

DATE __________

RISE: ______   BEDTIME: ______   SLEEP (HRS): ______

NOTES FOR THE DAY

IN A STATE OF KETOSIS?

YES   NO   UNSURE

WATER INTAKE TRACKER

EXERCISE / WORKOUT ROUTINE

DAILY ENERGY LEVEL

HIGH   **MEDIUM**   **LOW**

BREAKFAST

FAT: CARBS: PROTEIN: CALORIES:

LUNCH

FAT: CARBS: PROTEIN: CALORIES:

DINNER

FAT: CARBS: PROTEIN: CALORIES:

SNACKS

FAT: CARBS: PROTEIN: CALORIES:

HOW DO I FEEL TODAY?

TOP 6 PRIORITIES OF THE DAY

END OF THE DAY TOTAL OVERVIEW

CARBS   FAT   PROTEIN   CALORIES

DAILY PROGRESS TRACKER

SLEEP TRACKER:

DATE

RISE:

BEDTIME:

SLEEP (HRS):

NOTES FOR THE DAY

IN A STATE OF KETOSIS?

YES   NO   UNSURE

WATER INTAKE TRACKER

EXERCISE / WORKOUT ROUTINE

DAILY ENERGY LEVEL		
HIGH	MEDIUM	LOW

BREAKFAST

FAT: CARBS: PROTEIN: CALORIES:

LUNCH

FAT: CARBS: PROTEIN: CALORIES:

DINNER

FAT: CARBS: PROTEIN: CALORIES:

SNACKS

FAT: CARBS: PROTEIN: CALORIES:

HOW DO I FEEL TODAY?

TOP 6 PRIORITIES OF THE DAY

END OF THE DAY TOTAL OVERVIEW

CARBS   FAT   PROTEIN   CALORIES

DAILY PROGRESS TRACKER

SLEEP TRACKER:

DATE ______________

RISE: __________   BEDTIME: __________   SLEEP (HRS): __________

NOTES FOR THE DAY

____

____

EXERCISE / WORKOUT ROUTINE

HOW DO I FEEL TODAY?

TOP 6 PRIORITIES OF THE DAY

____

____

IN A STATE OF KETOSIS?

YES   NO   UNSURE

WATER INTAKE TRACKER

DAILY ENERGY LEVEL

HIGH   **MEDIUM**   **LOW**

BREAKFAST

FAT: CARBS: PROTEIN: CALORIES:

LUNCH

FAT: CARBS: PROTEIN: CALORIES:

DINNER

FAT: CARBS: PROTEIN: CALORIES:

SNACKS

FAT: CARBS: PROTEIN: CALORIES:

END OF THE DAY TOTAL OVERVIEW

CARBS   FAT   PROTEIN   CALORIES

DAILY PROGRESS TRACKER

SLEEP TRACKER:

RISE: BEDTIME: SLEEP (HRS):

DATE

NOTES FOR THE DAY

EXERCISE / WORKOUT ROUTINE

HOW DO I FEEL TODAY?

TOP 6 PRIORITIES OF THE DAY

IN A STATE OF KETOSIS?

YES   NO   UNSURE

WATER INTAKE TRACKER

DAILY ENERGY LEVEL		
HIGH	MEDIUM	LOW

BREAKFAST

FAT: CARBS: PROTEIN: CALORIES:

LUNCH

FAT: CARBS: PROTEIN: CALORIES:

DINNER

FAT: CARBS: PROTEIN: CALORIES:

SNACKS

FAT: CARBS: PROTEIN: CALORIES:

END OF THE DAY TOTAL OVERVIEW

CARBS   FAT   PROTEIN   CALORIES

ONE MONTH PROGRESS MEASUREMENTS

MONTHLY GOAL

DATE:

CHEST					
WAIST					
SHOULDERS					
UPPER ARM					
FOREARM					
CALF					
WEIGHT					
TOTAL WEIGHT LOSS >>					

MONTH TWO

IT'S ONLY ANOTHER 30
DAYS.
JUST DO IT FOR ONE DAY.
THEN DO IT FOR ONE DAY
AGAIN (AGAIN).

GOALS & ACCOMPLISHMENTS

MONTH JAN   FEB   MAR   APR   MAY   JUN   JUL   AUG   SEP   OCT   NOV   DEC

THIS MONTH'S GOALS

ACTION PLAN   M T W T F S S

WEEKLY GOALS

M

T

W

T

F

S

S

NOTES:

THOUGHTS

MEALS:	BREAKFAST	LUNCH	DINNER	SNACKS
M				
T				
W				
T				
F				
S				
S				

MONTHLY PROGRESS TRACKER

JAN FEB MAR APR MAY JUN JUL AUG SEP OCT NOV DEC

MON	TUE	WED	THU	FRI	SAT	SUN

WEIGHT LOSS MILESTONE TRACKER

CHEAT DAY TRACKER

WEEKLY DIET SUCCESS TRACKER & NOTES

WEEKLY FASTING TRACKER

Week Of: _______________

MONDAY

| Goal | 12 1 2 3 4 5 6 7 8 9 10 11 12 1 2 3 4 5 6 7 8 9 10 11 |
| Actual | 12 1 2 3 4 5 6 7 8 9 10 11 12 1 2 3 4 5 6 7 8 9 10 11 |

TUESDAY

| Goal | 12 1 2 3 4 5 6 7 8 9 10 11 12 1 2 3 4 5 6 7 8 9 10 11 |
| Actual | 12 1 2 3 4 5 6 7 8 9 10 11 12 1 2 3 4 5 6 7 8 9 10 11 |

WEDNESDAY

| Goal | 12 1 2 3 4 5 6 7 8 9 10 11 12 1 2 3 4 5 6 7 8 9 10 11 |
| Actual | 12 1 2 3 4 5 6 7 8 9 10 11 12 1 2 3 4 5 6 7 8 9 10 11 |

THURSDAY

| Goal | 12 1 2 3 4 5 6 7 8 9 10 11 12 1 2 3 4 5 6 7 8 9 10 11 |
| Actual | 12 1 2 3 4 5 6 7 8 9 10 11 12 1 2 3 4 5 6 7 8 9 10 11 |

FRIDAY

| Goal | 12 1 2 3 4 5 6 7 8 9 10 11 12 1 2 3 4 5 6 7 8 9 10 11 |
| Actual | 12 1 2 3 4 5 6 7 8 9 10 11 12 1 2 3 4 5 6 7 8 9 10 11 |

SATURDAY

| Goal | 12 1 2 3 4 5 6 7 8 9 10 11 12 1 2 3 4 5 6 7 8 9 10 11 |
| Actual | 12 1 2 3 4 5 6 7 8 9 10 11 12 1 2 3 4 5 6 7 8 9 10 11 |

SUNDAY

| Goal | 12 1 2 3 4 5 6 7 8 9 10 11 12 1 2 3 4 5 6 7 8 9 10 11 |
| Actual | 12 1 2 3 4 5 6 7 8 9 10 11 12 1 2 3 4 5 6 7 8 9 10 11 |

WEEKLY MEAL PLANNER

Week of: _______________

	Breakfast	Lunch	Dinner	Snack	Other
Monday	TOTAL Carbs Fat Protein Cals	TOTAL Carbs Fat Protein Cals	TOTAL Carbs Fat Protein Cals	TOTAL Carbs Fat Protein Cals	TOTAL Carbs Fat Protein Cals
Tuesday	TOTAL Carbs Fat Protein Cals	TOTAL Carbs Fat Protein Cals	TOTAL Carbs Fat Protein Cals	TOTAL Carbs Fat Protein Cals	TOTAL Carbs Fat Protein Cals
Wednesday	TOTAL Carbs Fat Protein Cals	TOTAL Carbs Fat Protein Cals	TOTAL Carbs Fat Protein Cals	TOTAL Carbs Fat Protein Cals	TOTAL Carbs Fat Protein Cals
Thursday	TOTAL Carbs Fat Protein Cals	TOTAL Carbs Fat Protein Cals	TOTAL Carbs Fat Protein Cals	TOTAL Carbs Fat Protein Cals	TOTAL Carbs Fat Protein Cals
Friday	TOTAL Carbs Fat Protein Cals	TOTAL Carbs Fat Protein Cals	TOTAL Carbs Fat Protein Cals	TOTAL Carbs Fat Protein Cals	TOTAL Carbs Fat Protein Cals
Saturday	TOTAL Carbs Fat Protein Cals	TOTAL Carbs Fat Protein Cals	TOTAL Carbs Fat Protein Cals	TOTAL Carbs Fat Protein Cals	TOTAL Carbs Fat Protein Cals
Sunday	TOTAL Carbs Fat Protein Cals	TOTAL Carbs Fat Protein Cals	TOTAL Carbs Fat Protein Cals	TOTAL Carbs Fat Protein Cals	TOTAL Carbs Fat Protein Cals

WEEKLY LOW CARB SHOPPING LIST

FRESH PRODUCE

MEAT AND SEAFOOD

DAIRY PRODUCTS

PANTRY ITEMS

FROZEN / OTHER

DAILY PROGRESS TRACKER

SLEEP TRACKER:

DATE

RISE: BEDTIME: SLEEP (HRS):

NOTES FOR THE DAY

IN A STATE OF KETOSIS?

YES   NO   UNSURE

WATER INTAKE TRACKER

EXERCISE / WORKOUT ROUTINE

DAILY ENERGY LEVEL

HIGH   MEDIUM   LOW

BREAKFAST

FAT: CARBS: PROTEIN: CALORIES:

LUNCH

FAT: CARBS: PROTEIN: CALORIES:

DINNER

FAT: CARBS: PROTEIN: CALORIES:

SNACKS

FAT: CARBS: PROTEIN: CALORIES:

HOW DO I FEEL TODAY?

TOP 6 PRIORITIES OF THE DAY

END OF THE DAY TOTAL OVERVIEW

CARBS   FAT   PROTEIN   CALORIES

DAILY PROGRESS TRACKER

SLEEP TRACKER:

DATE

RISE:

BEDTIME:

SLEEP (HRS):

NOTES FOR THE DAY

IN A STATE OF KETOSIS?

YES   NO   UNSURE

WATER INTAKE TRACKER

EXERCISE / WORKOUT ROUTINE

DAILY ENERGY LEVEL

HIGH   **MEDIUM**   **LOW**

BREAKFAST

FAT: CARBS: PROTEIN: CALORIES:

LUNCH

FAT: CARBS: PROTEIN: CALORIES:

DINNER

FAT: CARBS: PROTEIN: CALORIES:

SNACKS

FAT: CARBS: PROTEIN: CALORIES:

HOW DO I FEEL TODAY?

TOP 6 PRIORITIES OF THE DAY

END OF THE DAY TOTAL OVERVIEW

CARBS   FAT   PROTEIN   CALORIES

DAILY PROGRESS TRACKER

SLEEP TRACKER:

DATE __________

RISE: __________   BEDTIME: __________   SLEEP (HRS): __________

NOTES FOR THE DAY

IN A STATE OF KETOSIS?

YES   NO   UNSURE

WATER INTAKE TRACKER

EXERCISE / WORKOUT ROUTINE

DAILY ENERGY LEVEL

HIGH   **MEDIUM**   **LOW**

BREAKFAST

FAT: CARBS: PROTEIN: CALORIES:

LUNCH

FAT: CARBS: PROTEIN: CALORIES:

DINNER

FAT: CARBS: PROTEIN: CALORIES:

SNACKS

FAT: CARBS: PROTEIN: CALORIES:

HOW DO I FEEL TODAY?

TOP 6 PRIORITIES OF THE DAY

END OF THE DAY TOTAL OVERVIEW

CARBS   FAT   PROTEIN   CALORIES

DAILY PROGRESS TRACKER

SLEEP TRACKER:

DATE ______

RISE: __________   BEDTIME: __________   SLEEP (HRS): __________

NOTES FOR THE DAY

IN A STATE OF KETOSIS?

YES   NO   UNSURE

WATER INTAKE TRACKER

EXERCISE / WORKOUT ROUTINE

DAILY ENERGY LEVEL

HIGH   **MEDIUM**   **LOW**

BREAKFAST

FAT: CARBS: PROTEIN: CALORIES:

LUNCH

FAT: CARBS: PROTEIN: CALORIES:

HOW DO I FEEL TODAY?

DINNER

FAT: CARBS: PROTEIN: CALORIES:

SNACKS

FAT: CARBS: PROTEIN: CALORIES:

TOP 6 PRIORITIES OF THE DAY

END OF THE DAY TOTAL OVERVIEW

CARBS   FAT   PROTEIN   CALORIES

DAILY PROGRESS TRACKER

SLEEP TRACKER:

DATE

RISE:

BEDTIME:

SLEEP (HRS):

NOTES FOR THE DAY

IN A STATE OF KETOSIS?

YES   NO   UNSURE

WATER INTAKE TRACKER

EXERCISE / WORKOUT ROUTINE

DAILY ENERGY LEVEL

HIGH   **MEDIUM**   **LOW**

BREAKFAST

FAT: CARBS: PROTEIN: CALORIES:

LUNCH

FAT: CARBS: PROTEIN: CALORIES:

DINNER

FAT: CARBS: PROTEIN: CALORIES:

SNACKS

FAT: CARBS: PROTEIN: CALORIES:

HOW DO I FEEL TODAY?

TOP 6 PRIORITIES OF THE DAY

END OF THE DAY TOTAL OVERVIEW

CARBS   FAT   PROTEIN   CALORIES

DAILY PROGRESS TRACKER

SLEEP TRACKER:

RISE: | BEDTIME: | SLEEP (HRS):

DATE

NOTES FOR THE DAY

IN A STATE OF KETOSIS?

YES   NO   UNSURE

WATER INTAKE TRACKER

EXERCISE / WORKOUT ROUTINE

DAILY ENERGY LEVEL

HIGH   **MEDIUM**   **LOW**

BREAKFAST

FAT: CARBS: PROTEIN: CALORIES:

LUNCH

FAT: CARBS: PROTEIN: CALORIES:

HOW DO I FEEL TODAY?

DINNER

FAT: CARBS: PROTEIN: CALORIES:

SNACKS

FAT: CARBS: PROTEIN: CALORIES:

TOP 6 PRIORITIES OF THE DAY

END OF THE DAY TOTAL OVERVIEW

CARBS   FAT   PROTEIN   CALORIES

DAILY PROGRESS TRACKER

SLEEP TRACKER:

DATE ________________

RISE: ______

BEDTIME: ______

SLEEP (HRS): ______

NOTES FOR THE DAY

IN A STATE OF KETOSIS?

YES   NO   UNSURE

WATER INTAKE TRACKER

EXERCISE / WORKOUT ROUTINE

DAILY ENERGY LEVEL

HIGH   **MEDIUM**   **LOW**

BREAKFAST

FAT: CARBS: PROTEIN: CALORIES:

LUNCH

FAT: CARBS: PROTEIN: CALORIES:

DINNER

FAT: CARBS: PROTEIN: CALORIES:

SNACKS

FAT: CARBS: PROTEIN: CALORIES:

HOW DO I FEEL TODAY?

TOP 6 PRIORITIES OF THE DAY

END OF THE DAY TOTAL OVERVIEW

CARBS   FAT   PROTEIN   CALORIES

WEEKLY FASTING TRACKER

Week Of: ___________________

MONDAY

| Goal | 12 | 1 | 2 | 3 | 4 | 5 | 6 | 7 | 8 | 9 | 10 | 11 | 12 | 1 | 2 | 3 | 4 | 5 | 6 | 7 | 8 | 9 | 10 | 11 |
| Actual | 12 | 1 | 2 | 3 | 4 | 5 | 6 | 7 | 8 | 9 | 10 | 11 | 12 | 1 | 2 | 3 | 4 | 5 | 6 | 7 | 8 | 9 | 10 | 11 |

TUESDAY

| Goal | 12 | 1 | 2 | 3 | 4 | 5 | 6 | 7 | 8 | 9 | 10 | 11 | 12 | 1 | 2 | 3 | 4 | 5 | 6 | 7 | 8 | 9 | 10 | 11 |
| Actual | 12 | 1 | 2 | 3 | 4 | 5 | 6 | 7 | 8 | 9 | 10 | 11 | 12 | 1 | 2 | 3 | 4 | 5 | 6 | 7 | 8 | 9 | 10 | 11 |

WEDNESDAY

| Goal | 12 | 1 | 2 | 3 | 4 | 5 | 6 | 7 | 8 | 9 | 10 | 11 | 12 | 1 | 2 | 3 | 4 | 5 | 6 | 7 | 8 | 9 | 10 | 11 |
| Actual | 12 | 1 | 2 | 3 | 4 | 5 | 6 | 7 | 8 | 9 | 10 | 11 | 12 | 1 | 2 | 3 | 4 | 5 | 6 | 7 | 8 | 9 | 10 | 11 |

THURSDAY

| Goal | 12 | 1 | 2 | 3 | 4 | 5 | 6 | 7 | 8 | 9 | 10 | 11 | 12 | 1 | 2 | 3 | 4 | 5 | 6 | 7 | 8 | 9 | 10 | 11 |
| Actual | 12 | 1 | 2 | 3 | 4 | 5 | 6 | 7 | 8 | 9 | 10 | 11 | 12 | 1 | 2 | 3 | 4 | 5 | 6 | 7 | 8 | 9 | 10 | 11 |

FRIDAY

| Goal | 12 | 1 | 2 | 3 | 4 | 5 | 6 | 7 | 8 | 9 | 10 | 11 | 12 | 1 | 2 | 3 | 4 | 5 | 6 | 7 | 8 | 9 | 10 | 11 |
| Actual | 12 | 1 | 2 | 3 | 4 | 5 | 6 | 7 | 8 | 9 | 10 | 11 | 12 | 1 | 2 | 3 | 4 | 5 | 6 | 7 | 8 | 9 | 10 | 11 |

SATURDAY

| Goal | 12 | 1 | 2 | 3 | 4 | 5 | 6 | 7 | 8 | 9 | 10 | 11 | 12 | 1 | 2 | 3 | 4 | 5 | 6 | 7 | 8 | 9 | 10 | 11 |
| Actual | 12 | 1 | 2 | 3 | 4 | 5 | 6 | 7 | 8 | 9 | 10 | 11 | 12 | 1 | 2 | 3 | 4 | 5 | 6 | 7 | 8 | 9 | 10 | 11 |

SUNDAY

| Goal | 12 | 1 | 2 | 3 | 4 | 5 | 6 | 7 | 8 | 9 | 10 | 11 | 12 | 1 | 2 | 3 | 4 | 5 | 6 | 7 | 8 | 9 | 10 | 11 |
| Actual | 12 | 1 | 2 | 3 | 4 | 5 | 6 | 7 | 8 | 9 | 10 | 11 | 12 | 1 | 2 | 3 | 4 | 5 | 6 | 7 | 8 | 9 | 10 | 11 |

WEEKLY MEAL PLANNER

Week of: _______________

	Breakfast	Lunch	Dinner	Snack	Other
Monday	TOTAL · Carbs · Fat · Protein · Cals	TOTAL · Carbs · Fat · Protein · Cals	TOTAL · Carbs · Fat · Protein · Cals	TOTAL · Carbs · Fat · Protein · Cals	TOTAL · Carbs · Fat · Protein · Cals
Tuesday	TOTAL · Carbs · Fat · Protein · Cals	TOTAL · Carbs · Fat · Protein · Cals	TOTAL · Carbs · Fat · Protein · Cals	TOTAL · Carbs · Fat · Protein · Cals	TOTAL · Carbs · Fat · Protein · Cals
Wednesday	TOTAL · Carbs · Fat · Protein · Cals	TOTAL · Carbs · Fat · Protein · Cals	TOTAL · Carbs · Fat · Protein · Cals	TOTAL · Carbs · Fat · Protein · Cals	TOTAL · Carbs · Fat · Protein · Cals
Thursday	TOTAL · Carbs · Fat · Protein · Cals	TOTAL · Carbs · Fat · Protein · Cals	TOTAL · Carbs · Fat · Protein · Cals	TOTAL · Carbs · Fat · Protein · Cals	TOTAL · Carbs · Fat · Protein · Cals
Friday	TOTAL · Carbs · Fat · Protein · Cals	TOTAL · Carbs · Fat · Protein · Cals	TOTAL · Carbs · Fat · Protein · Cals	TOTAL · Carbs · Fat · Protein · Cals	TOTAL · Carbs · Fat · Protein · Cals
Saturday	TOTAL · Carbs · Fat · Protein · Cals	TOTAL · Carbs · Fat · Protein · Cals	TOTAL · Carbs · Fat · Protein · Cals	TOTAL · Carbs · Fat · Protein · Cals	TOTAL · Carbs · Fat · Protein · Cals
Sunday	TOTAL · Carbs · Fat · Protein · Cals	TOTAL · Carbs · Fat · Protein · Cals	TOTAL · Carbs · Fat · Protein · Cals	TOTAL · Carbs · Fat · Protein · Cals	TOTAL · Carbs · Fat · Protein · Cals

WEEKLY LOW CARB SHOPPING LIST

FRESH PRODUCE

MEAT AND SEAFOOD

DAIRY PRODUCTS

PANTRY ITEMS

FROZEN / OTHER

DAILY PROGRESS TRACKER

SLEEP TRACKER:

DATE

RISE:

BEDTIME:

SLEEP (HRS):

NOTES FOR THE DAY

IN A STATE OF KETOSIS?

YES   NO   UNSURE

WATER INTAKE TRACKER

EXERCISE / WORKOUT ROUTINE

DAILY ENERGY LEVEL

HIGH   MEDIUM   LOW

BREAKFAST

FAT: CARBS: PROTEIN: CALORIES:

LUNCH

FAT: CARBS: PROTEIN: CALORIES:

DINNER

FAT: CARBS: PROTEIN: CALORIES:

HOW DO I FEEL TODAY?

SNACKS

FAT: CARBS: PROTEIN: CALORIES:

TOP 6 PRIORITIES OF THE DAY

END OF THE DAY TOTAL OVERVIEW

CARBS   FAT   PROTEIN   CALORIES

DAILY PROGRESS TRACKER

SLEEP TRACKER:

DATE _______________

RISE: _______________   BEDTIME: _______________   SLEEP (HRS): _______________

NOTES FOR THE DAY

____

____

____

EXERCISE / WORKOUT ROUTINE

HOW DO I FEEL TODAY?

TOP 6 PRIORITIES OF THE DAY

____

____

IN A STATE OF KETOSIS?

YES   NO   UNSURE

WATER INTAKE TRACKER

DAILY ENERGY LEVEL

HIGH   **MEDIUM**   **LOW**

BREAKFAST

FAT: CARBS: PROTEIN: CALORIES:

LUNCH

FAT: CARBS: PROTEIN: CALORIES:

DINNER

FAT: CARBS: PROTEIN: CALORIES:

SNACKS

FAT: CARBS: PROTEIN: CALORIES:

END OF THE DAY TOTAL OVERVIEW

CARBS   FAT   PROTEIN   CALORIES

DAILY PROGRESS TRACKER

SLEEP TRACKER:

DATE

RISE:

BEDTIME:

SLEEP (HRS):

NOTES FOR THE DAY

IN A STATE OF KETOSIS?

YES   NO   UNSURE

WATER INTAKE TRACKER

EXERCISE / WORKOUT ROUTINE

DAILY ENERGY LEVEL

HIGH   **MEDIUM**   **LOW**

BREAKFAST

FAT: CARBS: PROTEIN: CALORIES:

LUNCH

FAT: CARBS: PROTEIN: CALORIES:

HOW DO I FEEL TODAY?

DINNER

FAT: CARBS: PROTEIN: CALORIES:

SNACKS

FAT: CARBS: PROTEIN: CALORIES:

TOP 6 PRIORITIES OF THE DAY

END OF THE DAY TOTAL OVERVIEW

CARBS   FAT   PROTEIN   CALORIES

DAILY PROGRESS TRACKER

SLEEP TRACKER:

DATE

RISE:

BEDTIME:

SLEEP (HRS):

NOTES FOR THE DAY

IN A STATE OF KETOSIS?

YES   NO   UNSURE

WATER INTAKE TRACKER

EXERCISE / WORKOUT ROUTINE

DAILY ENERGY LEVEL

HIGH   **MEDIUM**   **LOW**

BREAKFAST

FAT: CARBS: PROTEIN: CALORIES:

LUNCH

FAT: CARBS: PROTEIN: CALORIES:

DINNER

FAT: CARBS: PROTEIN: CALORIES:

SNACKS

FAT: CARBS: PROTEIN: CALORIES:

HOW DO I FEEL TODAY?

TOP 6 PRIORITIES OF THE DAY

END OF THE DAY TOTAL OVERVIEW

CARBS   FAT   PROTEIN   CALORIES

DAILY PROGRESS TRACKER

SLEEP TRACKER:

DATE ___________

RISE: _______   BEDTIME: _______   SLEEP (HRS): _______

NOTES FOR THE DAY

IN A STATE OF KETOSIS?

YES   NO   UNSURE

WATER INTAKE TRACKER

EXERCISE / WORKOUT ROUTINE

DAILY ENERGY LEVEL		
HIGH	MEDIUM	LOW

BREAKFAST

FAT: CARBS: PROTEIN: CALORIES:

LUNCH

FAT: CARBS: PROTEIN: CALORIES:

DINNER

FAT: CARBS: PROTEIN: CALORIES:

SNACKS

FAT: CARBS: PROTEIN: CALORIES:

HOW DO I FEEL TODAY?

TOP 6 PRIORITIES OF THE DAY

END OF THE DAY TOTAL OVERVIEW

CARBS   FAT   PROTEIN   CALORIES

DAILY PROGRESS TRACKER

SLEEP TRACKER:

DATE ___________

RISE: ___________   BEDTIME: ___________   SLEEP (HRS): ___________

NOTES FOR THE DAY

IN A STATE OF KETOSIS?

YES   NO   UNSURE

WATER INTAKE TRACKER

EXERCISE / WORKOUT ROUTINE

DAILY ENERGY LEVEL

HIGH   MEDIUM   LOW

BREAKFAST

FAT: CARBS: PROTEIN: CALORIES:

HOW DO I FEEL TODAY?

LUNCH

FAT: CARBS: PROTEIN: CALORIES:

DINNER

FAT: CARBS: PROTEIN: CALORIES:

SNACKS

FAT: CARBS: PROTEIN: CALORIES:

TOP 6 PRIORITIES OF THE DAY

END OF THE DAY TOTAL OVERVIEW

CARBS   FAT   PROTEIN   CALORIES

DAILY PROGRESS TRACKER

SLEEP TRACKER:

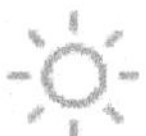 RISE:

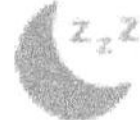 BEDTIME:

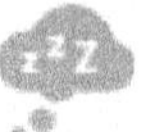 SLEEP (HRS):

NOTES FOR THE DAY

IN A STATE OF KETOSIS?

YES   NO   UNSURE

WATER INTAKE TRACKER

EXERCISE / WORKOUT ROUTINE

DAILY ENERGY LEVEL

HIGH   **MEDIUM**   **LOW**

BREAKFAST

FAT: CARBS: PROTEIN: CALORIES:

LUNCH

FAT: CARBS: PROTEIN: CALORIES:

DINNER

FAT: CARBS: PROTEIN: CALORIES:

HOW DO I FEEL TODAY?

SNACKS

FAT: CARBS: PROTEIN: CALORIES:

TOP 6 PRIORITIES OF THE DAY

END OF THE DAY TOTAL OVERVIEW

CARBS   FAT   PROTEIN   CALORIES

 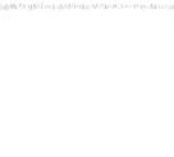  

WEEKLY FASTING TRACKER

Week Of: _______________

MONDAY

Goal	12	1	2	3	4	5	6	7	8	9	10	11	12	1	2	3	4	5	6	7	8	9	10	11
Actual	12	1	2	3	4	5	6	7	8	9	10	11	12	1	2	3	4	5	6	7	8	9	10	11

TUESDAY

Goal	12	1	2	3	4	5	6	7	8	9	10	11	12	1	2	3	4	5	6	7	8	9	10	11
Actual	12	1	2	3	4	5	6	7	8	9	10	11	12	1	2	3	4	5	6	7	8	9	10	11

WEDNESDAY

Goal	12	1	2	3	4	5	6	7	8	9	10	11	12	1	2	3	4	5	6	7	8	9	10	11
Actual	12	1	2	3	4	5	6	7	8	9	10	11	12	1	2	3	4	5	6	7	8	9	10	11

THURSDAY

Goal	12	1	2	3	4	5	6	7	8	9	10	11	12	1	2	3	4	5	6	7	8	9	10	11
Actual	12	1	2	3	4	5	6	7	8	9	10	11	12	1	2	3	4	5	6	7	8	9	10	11

FRIDAY

Goal	12	1	2	3	4	5	6	7	8	9	10	11	12	1	2	3	4	5	6	7	8	9	10	11
Actual	12	1	2	3	4	5	6	7	8	9	10	11	12	1	2	3	4	5	6	7	8	9	10	11

SATURDAY

Goal	12	1	2	3	4	5	6	7	8	9	10	11	12	1	2	3	4	5	6	7	8	9	10	11
Actual	12	1	2	3	4	5	6	7	8	9	10	11	12	1	2	3	4	5	6	7	8	9	10	11

SUNDAY

Goal	12	1	2	3	4	5	6	7	8	9	10	11	12	1	2	3	4	5	6	7	8	9	10	11
Actual	12	1	2	3	4	5	6	7	8	9	10	11	12	1	2	3	4	5	6	7	8	9	10	11

WEEKLY MEAL PLANNER

Week of: _______________

	Breakfast	Lunch	Dinner	Snack	Other
Monday	TOTAL Carbs Fat Protein Cals	TOTAL Carbs Fat Protein Cals	TOTAL Carbs Fat Protein Cals	TOTAL Carbs Fat Protein Cals	TOTAL Carbs Fat Protein Cals
Tuesday	TOTAL Carbs Fat Protein Cals	TOTAL Carbs Fat Protein Cals	TOTAL Carbs Fat Protein Cals	TOTAL Carbs Fat Protein Cals	TOTAL Carbs Fat Protein Cals
Wednesday	TOTAL Carbs Fat Protein Cals	TOTAL Carbs Fat Protein Cals	TOTAL Carbs Fat Protein Cals	TOTAL Carbs Fat Protein Cals	TOTAL Carbs Fat Protein Cals
Thursday	TOTAL Carbs Fat Protein Cals	TOTAL Carbs Fat Protein Cals	TOTAL Carbs Fat Protein Cals	TOTAL Carbs Fat Protein Cals	TOTAL Carbs Fat Protein Cals
Friday	TOTAL Carbs Fat Protein Cals	TOTAL Carbs Fat Protein Cals	TOTAL Carbs Fat Protein Cals	TOTAL Carbs Fat Protein Cals	TOTAL Carbs Fat Protein Cals
Saturday	TOTAL Carbs Fat Protein Cals	TOTAL Carbs Fat Protein Cals	TOTAL Carbs Fat Protein Cals	TOTAL Carbs Fat Protein Cals	TOTAL Carbs Fat Protein Cals
Sunday	TOTAL Carbs Fat Protein Cals	TOTAL Carbs Fat Protein Cals	TOTAL Carbs Fat Protein Cals	TOTAL Carbs Fat Protein Cals	TOTAL Carbs Fat Protein Cals

WEEKLY LOW CARB SHOPPING LIST

FRESH PRODUCE

MEAT AND SEAFOOD

DAIRY PRODUCTS

PANTRY ITEMS

FROZEN / OTHER

DAILY PROGRESS TRACKER

SLEEP TRACKER:

RISE: ___________   BEDTIME: ___________

DATE ___________

SLEEP (HRS): ___________

NOTES FOR THE DAY

IN A STATE OF KETOSIS?

YES   NO   UNSURE

WATER INTAKE TRACKER

EXERCISE / WORKOUT ROUTINE

DAILY ENERGY LEVEL

HIGH   MEDIUM   LOW

BREAKFAST

FAT: CARBS: PROTEIN: CALORIES:

LUNCH

FAT: CARBS: PROTEIN: CALORIES:

DINNER

FAT: CARBS: PROTEIN: CALORIES:

HOW DO I FEEL TODAY?

SNACKS

FAT: CARBS: PROTEIN: CALORIES:

TOP 6 PRIORITIES OF THE DAY

END OF THE DAY TOTAL OVERVIEW

CARBS   FAT   PROTEIN   CALORIES

DAILY PROGRESS TRACKER

SLEEP TRACKER:

DATE _______________

RISE: ______   BEDTIME: ______   SLEEP (HRS): ______

NOTES FOR THE DAY

IN A STATE OF KETOSIS?

YES   NO   UNSURE

WATER INTAKE TRACKER

EXERCISE / WORKOUT ROUTINE

DAILY ENERGY LEVEL

HIGH   **MEDIUM**   **LOW**

BREAKFAST

FAT: CARBS: PROTEIN: CALORIES:

LUNCH

FAT: CARBS: PROTEIN: CALORIES:

DINNER

FAT: CARBS: PROTEIN: CALORIES:

SNACKS

FAT: CARBS: PROTEIN: CALORIES:

HOW DO I FEEL TODAY?

TOP 6 PRIORITIES OF THE DAY

END OF THE DAY TOTAL OVERVIEW

CARBS   FAT   PROTEIN   CALORIES

DAILY PROGRESS TRACKER

SLEEP TRACKER:

DATE

RISE: BEDTIME: SLEEP (HRS):

NOTES FOR THE DAY

IN A STATE OF KETOSIS?

YES   NO   UNSURE

WATER INTAKE TRACKER

EXERCISE / WORKOUT ROUTINE

DAILY ENERGY LEVEL		
HIGH	MEDIUM	LOW

BREAKFAST

FAT: CARBS: PROTEIN: CALORIES:

LUNCH

FAT: CARBS: PROTEIN: CALORIES:

DINNER

FAT: CARBS: PROTEIN: CALORIES:

SNACKS

FAT: CARBS: PROTEIN: CALORIES:

HOW DO I FEEL TODAY?

TOP 6 PRIORITIES OF THE DAY

END OF THE DAY TOTAL OVERVIEW

CARBS   FAT   PROTEIN   CALORIES

DAILY PROGRESS TRACKER

SLEEP TRACKER:

DATE

RISE:

BEDTIME:

SLEEP (HRS):

NOTES FOR THE DAY

IN A STATE OF KETOSIS?

YES   NO   UNSURE

WATER INTAKE TRACKER

EXERCISE / WORKOUT ROUTINE

DAILY ENERGY LEVEL

HIGH   **MEDIUM**   **LOW**

BREAKFAST

FAT: CARBS: PROTEIN: CALORIES:

LUNCH

FAT: CARBS: PROTEIN: CALORIES:

DINNER

FAT: CARBS: PROTEIN: CALORIES:

SNACKS

FAT: CARBS: PROTEIN: CALORIES:

HOW DO I FEEL TODAY?

TOP 6 PRIORITIES OF THE DAY

END OF THE DAY TOTAL OVERVIEW

CARBS   FAT   PROTEIN   CALORIES

DAILY PROGRESS TRACKER

SLEEP TRACKER:

DATE

RISE:

BEDTIME:

SLEEP (HRS):

NOTES FOR THE DAY

IN A STATE OF KETOSIS?

YES   NO   UNSURE

WATER INTAKE TRACKER

EXERCISE / WORKOUT ROUTINE

DAILY ENERGY LEVEL

HIGH   MEDIUM   LOW

BREAKFAST

FAT: CARBS: PROTEIN: CALORIES:

HOW DO I FEEL TODAY?

LUNCH

FAT: CARBS: PROTEIN: CALORIES:

DINNER

FAT: CARBS: PROTEIN: CALORIES:

SNACKS

FAT: CARBS: PROTEIN: CALORIES:

TOP 6 PRIORITIES OF THE DAY

END OF THE DAY TOTAL OVERVIEW

CARBS   FAT   PROTEIN   CALORIES

DAILY PROGRESS TRACKER

SLEEP TRACKER:

DATE

RISE:

BEDTIME:

SLEEP (HRS):

NOTES FOR THE DAY

IN A STATE OF KETOSIS?

YES   NO   UNSURE

WATER INTAKE TRACKER

EXERCISE / WORKOUT ROUTINE

DAILY ENERGY LEVEL

HIGH   **MEDIUM**   **LOW**

BREAKFAST

FAT: CARBS: PROTEIN: CALORIES:

LUNCH

FAT: CARBS: PROTEIN: CALORIES:

HOW DO I FEEL TODAY?

DINNER

FAT: CARBS: PROTEIN: CALORIES:

SNACKS

FAT: CARBS: PROTEIN: CALORIES:

TOP 6 PRIORITIES OF THE DAY

END OF THE DAY TOTAL OVERVIEW

CARBS   FAT   PROTEIN   CALORIES

DAILY PROGRESS TRACKER

SLEEP TRACKER:

RISE: BEDTIME: SLEEP (HRS):

DATE _______________

NOTES FOR THE DAY

IN A STATE OF KETOSIS?

YES   NO   UNSURE

WATER INTAKE TRACKER

EXERCISE / WORKOUT ROUTINE

DAILY ENERGY LEVEL		
HIGH	MEDIUM	LOW

BREAKFAST

FAT: CARBS: PROTEIN: CALORIES:

LUNCH

FAT: CARBS: PROTEIN: CALORIES:

DINNER

FAT: CARBS: PROTEIN: CALORIES:

SNACKS

FAT: CARBS: PROTEIN: CALORIES:

HOW DO I FEEL TODAY?

TOP 6 PRIORITIES OF THE DAY

END OF THE DAY TOTAL OVERVIEW

CARBS   FAT   PROTEIN   CALORIES

WEEKLY FASTING TRACKER

Week Of: _______________________

MONDAY

Goal	12	1	2	3	4	5	6	7	8	9	10	11	12	1	2	3	4	5	6	7	8	9	10	11
Actual	12	1	2	3	4	5	6	7	8	9	10	11	12	1	2	3	4	5	6	7	8	9	10	11

TUESDAY

Goal	12	1	2	3	4	5	6	7	8	9	10	11	12	1	2	3	4	5	6	7	8	9	10	11
Actual	12	1	2	3	4	5	6	7	8	9	10	11	12	1	2	3	4	5	6	7	8	9	10	11

WEDNESDAY

Goal	12	1	2	3	4	5	6	7	8	9	10	11	12	1	2	3	4	5	6	7	8	9	10	11
Actual	12	1	2	3	4	5	6	7	8	9	10	11	12	1	2	3	4	5	6	7	8	9	10	11

THURSDAY

Goal	12	1	2	3	4	5	6	7	8	9	10	11	12	1	2	3	4	5	6	7	8	9	10	11
Actual	12	1	2	3	4	5	6	7	8	9	10	11	12	1	2	3	4	5	6	7	8	9	10	11

FRIDAY

Goal	12	1	2	3	4	5	6	7	8	9	10	11	12	1	2	3	4	5	6	7	8	9	10	11
Actual	12	1	2	3	4	5	6	7	8	9	10	11	12	1	2	3	4	5	6	7	8	9	10	11

SATURDAY

Goal	12	1	2	3	4	5	6	7	8	9	10	11	12	1	2	3	4	5	6	7	8	9	10	11
Actual	12	1	2	3	4	5	6	7	8	9	10	11	12	1	2	3	4	5	6	7	8	9	10	11

SUNDAY

Goal	12	1	2	3	4	5	6	7	8	9	10	11	12	1	2	3	4	5	6	7	8	9	10	11
Actual	12	1	2	3	4	5	6	7	8	9	10	11	12	1	2	3	4	5	6	7	8	9	10	11

WEEKLY MEAL PLANNER

Week of: _______________

	Breakfast	Lunch	Dinner	Snack	Other
Monday	TOTAL Carbs Fat Protein Cals	TOTAL Carbs Fat Protein Cals	TOTAL Carbs Fat Protein Cals	TOTAL Carbs Fat Protein Cals	TOTAL Carbs Fat Protein Cals
Tuesday	TOTAL Carbs Fat Protein Cals	TOTAL Carbs Fat Protein Cals	TOTAL Carbs Fat Protein Cals	TOTAL Carbs Fat Protein Cals	TOTAL Carbs Fat Protein Cals
Wednesday	TOTAL Carbs Fat Protein Cals	TOTAL Carbs Fat Protein Cals	TOTAL Carbs Fat Protein Cals	TOTAL Carbs Fat Protein Cals	TOTAL Carbs Fat Protein Cals
Thursday	TOTAL Carbs Fat Protein Cals	TOTAL Carbs Fat Protein Cals	TOTAL Carbs Fat Protein Cals	TOTAL Carbs Fat Protein Cals	TOTAL Carbs Fat Protein Cals
Friday	TOTAL Carbs Fat Protein Cals	TOTAL Carbs Fat Protein Cals	TOTAL Carbs Fat Protein Cals	TOTAL Carbs Fat Protein Cals	TOTAL Carbs Fat Protein Cals
Saturday	TOTAL Carbs Fat Protein Cals	TOTAL Carbs Fat Protein Cals	TOTAL Carbs Fat Protein Cals	TOTAL Carbs Fat Protein Cals	TOTAL Carbs Fat Protein Cals
Sunday	TOTAL Carbs Fat Protein Cals	TOTAL Carbs Fat Protein Cals	TOTAL Carbs Fat Protein Cals	TOTAL Carbs Fat Protein Cals	TOTAL Carbs Fat Protein Cals

WEEKLY LOW CARB SHOPPING LIST

FRESH PRODUCE

MEAT AND SEAFOOD

DAIRY PRODUCTS

PANTRY ITEMS

FROZEN / OTHER

DAILY PROGRESS TRACKER

SLEEP TRACKER:

DATE

RISE:

BEDTIME:

SLEEP (HRS):

NOTES FOR THE DAY

IN A STATE OF KETOSIS?

YES   NO   UNSURE

WATER INTAKE TRACKER

EXERCISE / WORKOUT ROUTINE

DAILY ENERGY LEVEL		
HIGH	**MEDIUM**	**LOW**

BREAKFAST

FAT: CARBS: PROTEIN: CALORIES:

LUNCH

FAT: CARBS: PROTEIN: CALORIES:

HOW DO I FEEL TODAY?

DINNER

FAT: CARBS: PROTEIN: CALORIES:

SNACKS

FAT: CARBS: PROTEIN: CALORIES:

TOP 6 PRIORITIES OF THE DAY

END OF THE DAY TOTAL OVERVIEW

CARBS   FAT   PROTEIN   CALORIES

DAILY PROGRESS TRACKER

SLEEP TRACKER:

DATE ___________

RISE: __________   BEDTIME: __________   SLEEP (HRS): __________

NOTES FOR THE DAY

____

____

IN A STATE OF KETOSIS?

YES   NO   UNSURE

WATER INTAKE TRACKER

EXERCISE / WORKOUT ROUTINE

DAILY ENERGY LEVEL

HIGH   MEDIUM   LOW

BREAKFAST

FAT: CARBS: PROTEIN: CALORIES:

LUNCH

FAT: CARBS: PROTEIN: CALORIES:

DINNER

FAT: CARBS: PROTEIN: CALORIES:

SNACKS

FAT: CARBS: PROTEIN: CALORIES:

HOW DO I FEEL TODAY?

TOP 6 PRIORITIES OF THE DAY

END OF THE DAY TOTAL OVERVIEW

CARBS   FAT   PROTEIN   CALORIES

DAILY PROGRESS TRACKER

SLEEP TRACKER:

 RISE: 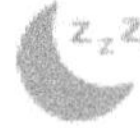 BEDTIME: 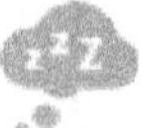 SLEEP (HRS):

NOTES FOR THE DAY

IN A STATE OF KETOSIS?

YES   NO   UNSURE

WATER INTAKE TRACKER

EXERCISE / WORKOUT ROUTINE

DAILY ENERGY LEVEL

HIGH   **MEDIUM**   **LOW**

BREAKFAST

FAT: CARBS: PROTEIN: CALORIES:

LUNCH

FAT: CARBS: PROTEIN: CALORIES:

DINNER

FAT: CARBS: PROTEIN: CALORIES:

HOW DO I FEEL TODAY?

SNACKS

FAT: CARBS: PROTEIN: CALORIES:

TOP 6 PRIORITIES OF THE DAY

END OF THE DAY TOTAL OVERVIEW

CARBS   FAT   PROTEIN   CALORIES

DAILY PROGRESS TRACKER

SLEEP TRACKER:

DATE ___________

RISE: | BEDTIME: | SLEEP (HRS):

NOTES FOR THE DAY

IN A STATE OF KETOSIS?

YES   NO   UNSURE

WATER INTAKE TRACKER

EXERCISE / WORKOUT ROUTINE

DAILY ENERGY LEVEL

HIGH   **MEDIUM**   **LOW**

BREAKFAST

FAT: CARBS: PROTEIN: CALORIES:

LUNCH

FAT: CARBS: PROTEIN: CALORIES:

DINNER

FAT: CARBS: PROTEIN: CALORIES:

SNACKS

FAT: CARBS: PROTEIN: CALORIES:

HOW DO I FEEL TODAY?

TOP 6 PRIORITIES OF THE DAY

END OF THE DAY TOTAL OVERVIEW

CARBS   FAT   PROTEIN   CALORIES

DAILY PROGRESS TRACKER

SLEEP TRACKER:

RISE: BEDTIME: SLEEP (HRS):

DATE

NOTES FOR THE DAY

IN A STATE OF KETOSIS?

YES   NO   UNSURE

WATER INTAKE TRACKER

EXERCISE / WORKOUT ROUTINE

DAILY ENERGY LEVEL

HIGH   **MEDIUM**   **LOW**

BREAKFAST

FAT: CARBS: PROTEIN: CALORIES:

LUNCH

FAT: CARBS: PROTEIN: CALORIES:

DINNER

FAT: CARBS: PROTEIN: CALORIES:

SNACKS

FAT: CARBS: PROTEIN: CALORIES:

HOW DO I FEEL TODAY?

TOP 6 PRIORITIES OF THE DAY

END OF THE DAY TOTAL OVERVIEW

CARBS   FAT   PROTEIN   CALORIES

DAILY PROGRESS TRACKER

SLEEP TRACKER:

DATE ____________

RISE: ____________ BEDTIME: ____________ SLEEP (HRS): ____________

NOTES FOR THE DAY

IN A STATE OF KETOSIS?

YES   NO   UNSURE

WATER INTAKE TRACKER

EXERCISE / WORKOUT ROUTINE

DAILY ENERGY LEVEL

HIGH   MEDIUM   LOW

BREAKFAST

FAT: CARBS: PROTEIN: CALORIES:

LUNCH

FAT: CARBS: PROTEIN: CALORIES:

DINNER

FAT: CARBS: PROTEIN: CALORIES:

SNACKS

FAT: CARBS: PROTEIN: CALORIES:

HOW DO I FEEL TODAY?

TOP 6 PRIORITIES OF THE DAY

END OF THE DAY TOTAL OVERVIEW

CARBS   FAT   PROTEIN   CALORIES

DAILY PROGRESS TRACKER

SLEEP TRACKER:

DATE ________________

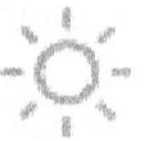 RISE: ____________

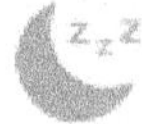 BEDTIME: ____________

 SLEEP (HRS): ____________

NOTES FOR THE DAY

IN A STATE OF KETOSIS?

YES   NO   UNSURE

WATER INTAKE TRACKER

EXERCISE / WORKOUT ROUTINE

DAILY ENERGY LEVEL

HIGH   **MEDIUM**   **LOW**

BREAKFAST

FAT: CARBS: PROTEIN: CALORIES:

LUNCH

FAT: CARBS: PROTEIN: CALORIES:

DINNER

FAT: CARBS: PROTEIN: CALORIES:

SNACKS

FAT: CARBS: PROTEIN: CALORIES:

HOW DO I FEEL TODAY?

TOP 6 PRIORITIES OF THE DAY

END OF THE DAY TOTAL OVERVIEW

CARBS   FAT   PROTEIN   CALORIES

TWO MONTH PROGRESS MEASUREMENTS

MONTHLY GOAL

DATE:

CHEST

WAIST

SHOULDERS

UPPER ARM

FOREARM

CALF

WEIGHT

TOTAL WEIGHT LOSS >>

MONTH THREE

YOU'RE ON THE HOME STRETCH.
IT'S ONLY ANOTHER 30 DAYS.
JUST DO IT FOR ONE DAY.
THEN DO IT FOR ONE DAY AGAIN (AGAIN).

GOALS & ACCOMPLISHMENTS

MONTH JAN FEB MAR APR MAY JUN JUL AUG SEP OCT NOV DEC

THIS MONTH'S GOALS

ACTION PLAN   M T W T F S S

WEEKLY GOALS

M
T
W
T
F
S
S

NOTES:

THOUGHTS

MEALS:	BREAKFAST	LUNCH	DINNER	SNACKS
M				
T				
W				
T				
F				
S				
S				

MONTHLY PROGRESS TRACKER

JAN FEB MAR APR MAY JUN JUL AUG SEP OCT NOV DEC

MON	TUE	WED	THU	FRI	SAT	SUN

WEIGHT LOSS MILESTONE TRACKER

CHEAT DAY TRACKER

WEEKLY DIET SUCCESS TRACKER & NOTES

WEEKLY FASTING TRACKER

Week Of: _______________________

MONDAY

Goal	12	1	2	3	4	5	6	7	8	9	10	11	12	1	2	3	4	5	6	7	8	9	10	11
Actual	12	1	2	3	4	5	6	7	8	9	10	11	12	1	2	3	4	5	6	7	8	9	10	11

TUESDAY

Goal	12	1	2	3	4	5	6	7	8	9	10	11	12	1	2	3	4	5	6	7	8	9	10	11
Actual	12	1	2	3	4	5	6	7	8	9	10	11	12	1	2	3	4	5	6	7	8	9	10	11

WEDNESDAY

Goal	12	1	2	3	4	5	6	7	8	9	10	11	12	1	2	3	4	5	6	7	8	9	10	11
Actual	12	1	2	3	4	5	6	7	8	9	10	11	12	1	2	3	4	5	6	7	8	9	10	11

THURSDAY

Goal	12	1	2	3	4	5	6	7	8	9	10	11	12	1	2	3	4	5	6	7	8	9	10	11
Actual	12	1	2	3	4	5	6	7	8	9	10	11	12	1	2	3	4	5	6	7	8	9	10	11

FRIDAY

Goal	12	1	2	3	4	5	6	7	8	9	10	11	12	1	2	3	4	5	6	7	8	9	10	11
Actual	12	1	2	3	4	5	6	7	8	9	10	11	12	1	2	3	4	5	6	7	8	9	10	11

SATURDAY

Goal	12	1	2	3	4	5	6	7	8	9	10	11	12	1	2	3	4	5	6	7	8	9	10	11
Actual	12	1	2	3	4	5	6	7	8	9	10	11	12	1	2	3	4	5	6	7	8	9	10	11

SUNDAY

Goal	12	1	2	3	4	5	6	7	8	9	10	11	12	1	2	3	4	5	6	7	8	9	10	11
Actual	12	1	2	3	4	5	6	7	8	9	10	11	12	1	2	3	4	5	6	7	8	9	10	11

WEEKLY MEAL PLANNER

Week of: _______________

	Breakfast	Lunch	Dinner	Snack	Other
Monday	Carbs Fat Protein Cals TOTAL	Carbs Fat Protein Cals TOTAL	Carbs Fat Protein Cals TOTAL	Carbs Fat Protein Cals TOTAL	Carbs Fat Protein Cals TOTAL
Tuesday	Carbs Fat Protein Cals TOTAL	Carbs Fat Protein Cals TOTAL	Carbs Fat Protein Cals TOTAL	Carbs Fat Protein Cals TOTAL	Carbs Fat Protein Cals TOTAL
Wednesday	Carbs Fat Protein Cals TOTAL	Carbs Fat Protein Cals TOTAL	Carbs Fat Protein Cals TOTAL	Carbs Fat Protein Cals TOTAL	Carbs Fat Protein Cals TOTAL
Thursday	Carbs Fat Protein Cals TOTAL	Carbs Fat Protein Cals TOTAL	Carbs Fat Protein Cals TOTAL	Carbs Fat Protein Cals TOTAL	Carbs Fat Protein Cals TOTAL
Friday	Carbs Fat Protein Cals TOTAL	Carbs Fat Protein Cals TOTAL	Carbs Fat Protein Cals TOTAL	Carbs Fat Protein Cals TOTAL	Carbs Fat Protein Cals TOTAL
Saturday	Carbs Fat Protein Cals TOTAL	Carbs Fat Protein Cals TOTAL	Carbs Fat Protein Cals TOTAL	Carbs Fat Protein Cals TOTAL	Carbs Fat Protein Cals TOTAL
Sunday	Carbs Fat Protein Cals TOTAL	Carbs Fat Protein Cals TOTAL	Carbs Fat Protein Cals TOTAL	Carbs Fat Protein Cals TOTAL	Carbs Fat Protein Cals TOTAL

WEEKLY LOW CARB SHOPPING LIST

FRESH PRODUCE

MEAT AND SEAFOOD

DAIRY PRODUCTS

PANTRY ITEMS

FROZEN / OTHER

DAILY PROGRESS TRACKER

SLEEP TRACKER:

DATE ______________

RISE: | BEDTIME: | SLEEP (HRS):

NOTES FOR THE DAY

IN A STATE OF KETOSIS?

YES   NO   UNSURE

WATER INTAKE TRACKER

EXERCISE / WORKOUT ROUTINE

DAILY ENERGY LEVEL		
HIGH	MEDIUM	LOW

BREAKFAST

FAT: CARBS: PROTEIN: CALORIES:

LUNCH

FAT: CARBS: PROTEIN: CALORIES:

DINNER

FAT: CARBS: PROTEIN: CALORIES:

SNACKS

FAT: CARBS: PROTEIN: CALORIES:

HOW DO I FEEL TODAY?

TOP 6 PRIORITIES OF THE DAY

END OF THE DAY TOTAL OVERVIEW

CARBS   FAT   PROTEIN   CALORIES

DAILY PROGRESS TRACKER

SLEEP TRACKER:

DATE ________________

RISE: ____________   BEDTIME: ____________   SLEEP (HRS): ____________

NOTES FOR THE DAY

____

____

____

IN A STATE OF KETOSIS?

YES   NO   UNSURE

WATER INTAKE TRACKER

EXERCISE / WORKOUT ROUTINE

DAILY ENERGY LEVEL

HIGH   **MEDIUM**   **LOW**

BREAKFAST

FAT: CARBS: PROTEIN: CALORIES:

LUNCH

FAT: CARBS: PROTEIN: CALORIES:

DINNER

FAT: CARBS: PROTEIN: CALORIES:

SNACKS

FAT: CARBS: PROTEIN: CALORIES:

HOW DO I FEEL TODAY?

TOP 6 PRIORITIES OF THE DAY

END OF THE DAY TOTAL OVERVIEW

CARBS   FAT   PROTEIN   CALORIES

DAILY PROGRESS TRACKER

SLEEP TRACKER:

DATE _______________

RISE: ___________   BEDTIME: ___________   SLEEP (HRS): ___________

NOTES FOR THE DAY

____

____

____

IN A STATE OF KETOSIS?

YES   NO   UNSURE

WATER INTAKE TRACKER

EXERCISE / WORKOUT ROUTINE

DAILY ENERGY LEVEL

HIGH   **MEDIUM**   **LOW**

BREAKFAST

FAT: CARBS: PROTEIN: CALORIES:

LUNCH

FAT: CARBS: PROTEIN: CALORIES:

DINNER

FAT: CARBS: PROTEIN: CALORIES:

SNACKS

FAT: CARBS: PROTEIN: CALORIES:

HOW DO I FEEL TODAY?

TOP 6 PRIORITIES OF THE DAY

END OF THE DAY TOTAL OVERVIEW

CARBS   FAT   PROTEIN   CALORIES

DAILY PROGRESS TRACKER

SLEEP TRACKER:

DATE

RISE:

BEDTIME:

SLEEP (HRS):

NOTES FOR THE DAY

IN A STATE OF KETOSIS?

YES　　　NO　　　UNSURE

WATER INTAKE TRACKER

EXERCISE / WORKOUT ROUTINE

DAILY ENERGY LEVEL

HIGH　　　**MEDIUM**　　　**LOW**

BREAKFAST

FAT:　　CARBS:　　PROTEIN:　　CALORIES:

LUNCH

FAT:　　CARBS:　　PROTEIN:　　CALORIES:

DINNER

FAT:　　CARBS:　　PROTEIN:　　CALORIES:

SNACKS

FAT:　　CARBS:　　PROTEIN:　　CALORIES:

HOW DO I FEEL TODAY?

TOP 6 PRIORITIES OF THE DAY

END OF THE DAY TOTAL OVERVIEW

CARBS　　　FAT　　　PROTEIN　　　CALORIES

DAILY PROGRESS TRACKER

SLEEP TRACKER:

DATE ________________

 RISE: | 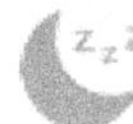 BEDTIME: | 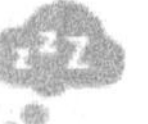 SLEEP (HRS):

NOTES FOR THE DAY

IN A STATE OF KETOSIS?

YES   NO   UNSURE

WATER INTAKE TRACKER

EXERCISE / WORKOUT ROUTINE

DAILY ENERGY LEVEL

HIGH   MEDIUM   LOW

BREAKFAST

FAT: CARBS: PROTEIN: CALORIES:

LUNCH

FAT: CARBS: PROTEIN: CALORIES:

DINNER

FAT: CARBS: PROTEIN: CALORIES:

SNACKS

FAT: CARBS: PROTEIN: CALORIES:

HOW DO I FEEL TODAY?

TOP 6 PRIORITIES OF THE DAY

END OF THE DAY TOTAL OVERVIEW

CARBS   FAT   PROTEIN   CALORIES

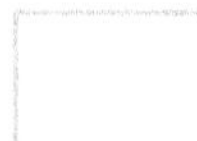 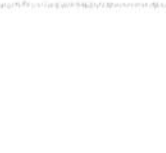 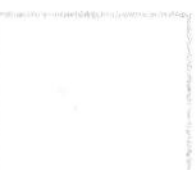 

DAILY PROGRESS TRACKER

SLEEP TRACKER:

DATE ___________

RISE: | BEDTIME: | SLEEP (HRS):

NOTES FOR THE DAY

IN A STATE OF KETOSIS?

YES   NO   UNSURE

WATER INTAKE TRACKER

EXERCISE / WORKOUT ROUTINE

DAILY ENERGY LEVEL

HIGH   **MEDIUM**   **LOW**

BREAKFAST

FAT: CARBS: PROTEIN: CALORIES:

LUNCH

FAT: CARBS: PROTEIN: CALORIES:

DINNER

FAT: CARBS: PROTEIN: CALORIES:

SNACKS

FAT: CARBS: PROTEIN: CALORIES:

HOW DO I FEEL TODAY?

TOP 6 PRIORITIES OF THE DAY

END OF THE DAY TOTAL OVERVIEW

CARBS   FAT   PROTEIN   CALORIES

DAILY PROGRESS TRACKER

SLEEP TRACKER:

DATE ____________

RISE: ____________ BEDTIME: ____________ SLEEP (HRS): ____________

NOTES FOR THE DAY

IN A STATE OF KETOSIS?

YES   NO   UNSURE

WATER INTAKE TRACKER

EXERCISE / WORKOUT ROUTINE

DAILY ENERGY LEVEL

HIGH   MEDIUM   LOW

BREAKFAST

FAT: CARBS: PROTEIN: CALORIES:

LUNCH

FAT: CARBS: PROTEIN: CALORIES:

DINNER

FAT: CARBS: PROTEIN: CALORIES:

SNACKS

FAT: CARBS: PROTEIN: CALORIES:

HOW DO I FEEL TODAY?

TOP 6 PRIORITIES OF THE DAY

END OF THE DAY TOTAL OVERVIEW

CARBS   FAT   PROTEIN   CALORIES

WEEKLY FASTING TRACKER

Week Of: _______________

MONDAY

Goal	12	1	2	3	4	5	6	7	8	9	10	11	12	1	2	3	4	5	6	7	8	9	10	11
Actual	12	1	2	3	4	5	6	7	8	9	10	11	12	1	2	3	4	5	6	7	8	9	10	11

TUESDAY

Goal	12	1	2	3	4	5	6	7	8	9	10	11	12	1	2	3	4	5	6	7	8	9	10	11
Actual	12	1	2	3	4	5	6	7	8	9	10	11	12	1	2	3	4	5	6	7	8	9	10	11

WEDNESDAY

Goal	12	1	2	3	4	5	6	7	8	9	10	11	12	1	2	3	4	5	6	7	8	9	10	11
Actual	12	1	2	3	4	5	6	7	8	9	10	11	12	1	2	3	4	5	6	7	8	9	10	11

THURSDAY

Goal	12	1	2	3	4	5	6	7	8	9	10	11	12	1	2	3	4	5	6	7	8	9	10	11
Actual	12	1	2	3	4	5	6	7	8	9	10	11	12	1	2	3	4	5	6	7	8	9	10	11

FRIDAY

Goal	12	1	2	3	4	5	6	7	8	9	10	11	12	1	2	3	4	5	6	7	8	9	10	11
Actual	12	1	2	3	4	5	6	7	8	9	10	11	12	1	2	3	4	5	6	7	8	9	10	11

SATURDAY

Goal	12	1	2	3	4	5	6	7	8	9	10	11	12	1	2	3	4	5	6	7	8	9	10	11
Actual	12	1	2	3	4	5	6	7	8	9	10	11	12	1	2	3	4	5	6	7	8	9	10	11

SUNDAY

Goal	12	1	2	3	4	5	6	7	8	9	10	11	12	1	2	3	4	5	6	7	8	9	10	11
Actual	12	1	2	3	4	5	6	7	8	9	10	11	12	1	2	3	4	5	6	7	8	9	10	11

WEEKLY MEAL PLANNER

Week of: _______________

	Breakfast	Lunch	Dinner	Snack	Other
Monday	Carbs Fat Protein Cals TOTAL	Carbs Fat Protein Cals TOTAL	Carbs Fat Protein Cals TOTAL	Carbs Fat Protein Cals TOTAL	Carbs Fat Protein Cals TOTAL
Tuesday	Carbs Fat Protein Cals TOTAL	Carbs Fat Protein Cals TOTAL	Carbs Fat Protein Cals TOTAL	Carbs Fat Protein Cals TOTAL	Carbs Fat Protein Cals TOTAL
Wednesday	Carbs Fat Protein Cals TOTAL	Carbs Fat Protein Cals TOTAL	Carbs Fat Protein Cals TOTAL	Carbs Fat Protein Cals TOTAL	Carbs Fat Protein Cals TOTAL
Thursday	Carbs Fat Protein Cals TOTAL	Carbs Fat Protein Cals TOTAL	Carbs Fat Protein Cals TOTAL	Carbs Fat Protein Cals TOTAL	Carbs Fat Protein Cals TOTAL
Friday	Carbs Fat Protein Cals TOTAL	Carbs Fat Protein Cals TOTAL	Carbs Fat Protein Cals TOTAL	Carbs Fat Protein Cals TOTAL	Carbs Fat Protein Cals TOTAL
Saturday	Carbs Fat Protein Cals TOTAL	Carbs Fat Protein Cals TOTAL	Carbs Fat Protein Cals TOTAL	Carbs Fat Protein Cals TOTAL	Carbs Fat Protein Cals TOTAL
Sunday	Carbs Fat Protein Cals TOTAL	Carbs Fat Protein Cals TOTAL	Carbs Fat Protein Cals TOTAL	Carbs Fat Protein Cals TOTAL	Carbs Fat Protein Cals TOTAL

WEEKLY LOW CARB SHOPPING LIST

FRESH PRODUCE

MEAT AND SEAFOOD

DAIRY PRODUCTS

PANTRY ITEMS

FROZEN / OTHER

DAILY PROGRESS TRACKER

SLEEP TRACKER:

DATE

RISE: BEDTIME: SLEEP (HRS):

NOTES FOR THE DAY

IN A STATE OF KETOSIS?

YES   NO   UNSURE

WATER INTAKE TRACKER

EXERCISE / WORKOUT ROUTINE

DAILY ENERGY LEVEL

HIGH   **MEDIUM**   **LOW**

BREAKFAST

FAT: CARBS: PROTEIN: CALORIES:

LUNCH

FAT: CARBS: PROTEIN: CALORIES:

DINNER

FAT: CARBS: PROTEIN: CALORIES:

SNACKS

FAT: CARBS: PROTEIN: CALORIES:

HOW DO I FEEL TODAY?

TOP 6 PRIORITIES OF THE DAY

END OF THE DAY TOTAL OVERVIEW

CARBS   FAT   PROTEIN   CALORIES

DAILY PROGRESS TRACKER

SLEEP TRACKER:

DATE ___________

RISE: __________   BEDTIME: __________   SLEEP (HRS): __________

NOTES FOR THE DAY

IN A STATE OF KETOSIS?

YES   NO   UNSURE

WATER INTAKE TRACKER

EXERCISE / WORKOUT ROUTINE

DAILY ENERGY LEVEL

HIGH   **MEDIUM**   **LOW**

BREAKFAST

FAT: CARBS: PROTEIN: CALORIES:

LUNCH

FAT: CARBS: PROTEIN: CALORIES:

DINNER

FAT: CARBS: PROTEIN: CALORIES:

SNACKS

FAT: CARBS: PROTEIN: CALORIES:

HOW DO I FEEL TODAY?

TOP 6 PRIORITIES OF THE DAY

END OF THE DAY TOTAL OVERVIEW

CARBS   FAT   PROTEIN   CALORIES

DAILY PROGRESS TRACKER

SLEEP TRACKER:

DATE

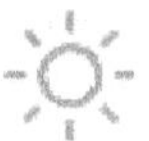 RISE:

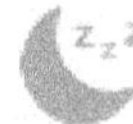 BEDTIME:

 SLEEP (HRS):

NOTES FOR THE DAY

IN A STATE OF KETOSIS?

YES NO UNSURE

WATER INTAKE TRACKER

EXERCISE / WORKOUT ROUTINE

DAILY ENERGY LEVEL

HIGH **MEDIUM** **LOW**

BREAKFAST

FAT: CARBS: PROTEIN: CALORIES:

LUNCH

FAT: CARBS: PROTEIN: CALORIES:

DINNER

FAT: CARBS: PROTEIN: CALORIES:

SNACKS

FAT: CARBS: PROTEIN: CALORIES:

HOW DO I FEEL TODAY?

TOP 6 PRIORITIES OF THE DAY

END OF THE DAY TOTAL OVERVIEW

CARBS FAT PROTEIN CALORIES

DAILY PROGRESS TRACKER

SLEEP TRACKER:

DATE _______________

RISE: _______   BEDTIME: _______   SLEEP (HRS): _______

NOTES FOR THE DAY

IN A STATE OF KETOSIS?

YES   NO   UNSURE

WATER INTAKE TRACKER

EXERCISE / WORKOUT ROUTINE

DAILY ENERGY LEVEL		
HIGH	**MEDIUM**	**LOW**

BREAKFAST

FAT: CARBS: PROTEIN: CALORIES:

LUNCH

FAT: CARBS: PROTEIN: CALORIES:

DINNER

FAT: CARBS: PROTEIN: CALORIES:

SNACKS

FAT: CARBS: PROTEIN: CALORIES:

HOW DO I FEEL TODAY?

TOP 6 PRIORITIES OF THE DAY

END OF THE DAY TOTAL OVERVIEW

CARBS   FAT   PROTEIN   CALORIES

DAILY PROGRESS TRACKER

SLEEP TRACKER:

DATE

RISE:

BEDTIME:

SLEEP (HRS):

NOTES FOR THE DAY

IN A STATE OF KETOSIS?

YES   NO   UNSURE

WATER INTAKE TRACKER

EXERCISE / WORKOUT ROUTINE

DAILY ENERGY LEVEL

HIGH   **MEDIUM**   **LOW**

BREAKFAST

FAT: CARBS: PROTEIN: CALORIES:

LUNCH

FAT: CARBS: PROTEIN: CALORIES:

HOW DO I FEEL TODAY?

DINNER

FAT: CARBS: PROTEIN: CALORIES:

SNACKS

FAT: CARBS: PROTEIN: CALORIES:

TOP 6 PRIORITIES OF THE DAY

END OF THE DAY TOTAL OVERVIEW

CARBS   FAT   PROTEIN   CALORIES

DAILY PROGRESS TRACKER

SLEEP TRACKER:

RISE: BEDTIME: SLEEP (HRS):

DATE

NOTES FOR THE DAY

EXERCISE / WORKOUT ROUTINE

HOW DO I FEEL TODAY?

TOP 6 PRIORITIES OF THE DAY

IN A STATE OF KETOSIS?

YES NO UNSURE

WATER INTAKE TRACKER

DAILY ENERGY LEVEL

HIGH MEDIUM LOW

BREAKFAST

FAT: CARBS: PROTEIN: CALORIES:

LUNCH

FAT: CARBS: PROTEIN: CALORIES:

DINNER

FAT: CARBS: PROTEIN: CALORIES:

SNACKS

FAT: CARBS: PROTEIN: CALORIES:

END OF THE DAY TOTAL OVERVIEW

CARBS FAT PROTEIN CALORIES

DAILY PROGRESS TRACKER

SLEEP TRACKER:

DATE ______________

RISE: | BEDTIME: | SLEEP (HRS):

NOTES FOR THE DAY

IN A STATE OF KETOSIS?

YES   NO   UNSURE

WATER INTAKE TRACKER

EXERCISE / WORKOUT ROUTINE

DAILY ENERGY LEVEL

HIGH   MEDIUM   LOW

BREAKFAST

FAT: CARBS: PROTEIN: CALORIES:

LUNCH

FAT: CARBS: PROTEIN: CALORIES:

DINNER

FAT: CARBS: PROTEIN: CALORIES:

SNACKS

FAT: CARBS: PROTEIN: CALORIES:

HOW DO I FEEL TODAY?

TOP 6 PRIORITIES OF THE DAY

END OF THE DAY TOTAL OVERVIEW

CARBS   FAT   PROTEIN   CALORIES

WEEKLY FASTING TRACKER

Week Of: _______________

MONDAY

Goal	12	1	2	3	4	5	6	7	8	9	10	11	12	1	2	3	4	5	6	7	8	9	10	11
Actual	12	1	2	3	4	5	6	7	8	9	10	11	12	1	2	3	4	5	6	7	8	9	10	11

TUESDAY

Goal	12	1	2	3	4	5	6	7	8	9	10	11	12	1	2	3	4	5	6	7	8	9	10	11
Actual	12	1	2	3	4	5	6	7	8	9	10	11	12	1	2	3	4	5	6	7	8	9	10	11

WEDNESDAY

Goal	12	1	2	3	4	5	6	7	8	9	10	11	12	1	2	3	4	5	6	7	8	9	10	11
Actual	12	1	2	3	4	5	6	7	8	9	10	11	12	1	2	3	4	5	6	7	8	9	10	11

THURSDAY

Goal	12	1	2	3	4	5	6	7	8	9	10	11	12	1	2	3	4	5	6	7	8	9	10	11
Actual	12	1	2	3	4	5	6	7	8	9	10	11	12	1	2	3	4	5	6	7	8	9	10	11

FRIDAY

Goal	12	1	2	3	4	5	6	7	8	9	10	11	12	1	2	3	4	5	6	7	8	9	10	11
Actual	12	1	2	3	4	5	6	7	8	9	10	11	12	1	2	3	4	5	6	7	8	9	10	11

SATURDAY

Goal	12	1	2	3	4	5	6	7	8	9	10	11	12	1	2	3	4	5	6	7	8	9	10	11
Actual	12	1	2	3	4	5	6	7	8	9	10	11	12	1	2	3	4	5	6	7	8	9	10	11

SUNDAY

Goal	12	1	2	3	4	5	6	7	8	9	10	11	12	1	2	3	4	5	6	7	8	9	10	11
Actual	12	1	2	3	4	5	6	7	8	9	10	11	12	1	2	3	4	5	6	7	8	9	10	11

WEEKLY MEAL PLANNER

Week of: ________________

	Breakfast	Lunch	Dinner	Snack	Other
Monday	TOTAL Carbs Fat Protein Cals	TOTAL Carbs Fat Protein Cals	TOTAL Carbs Fat Protein Cals	TOTAL Carbs Fat Protein Cals	TOTAL Carbs Fat Protein Cals
Tuesday	TOTAL Carbs Fat Protein Cals	TOTAL Carbs Fat Protein Cals	TOTAL Carbs Fat Protein Cals	TOTAL Carbs Fat Protein Cals	TOTAL Carbs Fat Protein Cals
Wednesday	TOTAL Carbs Fat Protein Cals	TOTAL Carbs Fat Protein Cals	TOTAL Carbs Fat Protein Cals	TOTAL Carbs Fat Protein Cals	TOTAL Carbs Fat Protein Cals
Thursday	TOTAL Carbs Fat Protein Cals	TOTAL Carbs Fat Protein Cals	TOTAL Carbs Fat Protein Cals	TOTAL Carbs Fat Protein Cals	TOTAL Carbs Fat Protein Cals
Friday	TOTAL Carbs Fat Protein Cals	TOTAL Carbs Fat Protein Cals	TOTAL Carbs Fat Protein Cals	TOTAL Carbs Fat Protein Cals	TOTAL Carbs Fat Protein Cals
Saturday	TOTAL Carbs Fat Protein Cals	TOTAL Carbs Fat Protein Cals	TOTAL Carbs Fat Protein Cals	TOTAL Carbs Fat Protein Cals	TOTAL Carbs Fat Protein Cals
Sunday	TOTAL Carbs Fat Protein Cals	TOTAL Carbs Fat Protein Cals	TOTAL Carbs Fat Protein Cals	TOTAL Carbs Fat Protein Cals	TOTAL Carbs Fat Protein Cals

WEEKLY LOW CARB SHOPPING LIST

FRESH PRODUCE

MEAT AND SEAFOOD

DAIRY PRODUCTS

PANTRY ITEMS

FROZEN / OTHER

DAILY PROGRESS TRACKER

SLEEP TRACKER:

DATE ___________

RISE: ___________ BEDTIME: ___________ SLEEP (HRS): ___________

NOTES FOR THE DAY

IN A STATE OF KETOSIS?

YES   NO   UNSURE

WATER INTAKE TRACKER

EXERCISE / WORKOUT ROUTINE

DAILY ENERGY LEVEL

HIGH   MEDIUM   LOW

BREAKFAST

FAT: CARBS: PROTEIN: CALORIES:

LUNCH

FAT: CARBS: PROTEIN: CALORIES:

DINNER

FAT: CARBS: PROTEIN: CALORIES:

SNACKS

FAT: CARBS: PROTEIN: CALORIES:

HOW DO I FEEL TODAY?

TOP 6 PRIORITIES OF THE DAY

END OF THE DAY TOTAL OVERVIEW

CARBS   FAT   PROTEIN   CALORIES

DAILY PROGRESS TRACKER

SLEEP TRACKER:

RISE: ___________

BEDTIME: ___________

SLEEP (HRS): ___________

DATE ___________

NOTES FOR THE DAY

EXERCISE / WORKOUT ROUTINE

HOW DO I FEEL TODAY?

TOP 6 PRIORITIES OF THE DAY

IN A STATE OF KETOSIS?

YES   NO   UNSURE

WATER INTAKE TRACKER

DAILY ENERGY LEVEL

HIGH   MEDIUM   LOW

BREAKFAST

FAT: CARBS: PROTEIN: CALORIES:

LUNCH

FAT: CARBS: PROTEIN: CALORIES:

DINNER

FAT: CARBS: PROTEIN: CALORIES:

SNACKS

FAT: CARBS: PROTEIN: CALORIES:

END OF THE DAY TOTAL OVERVIEW

CARBS   FAT   PROTEIN   CALORIES

DAILY PROGRESS TRACKER

SLEEP TRACKER:

RISE: BEDTIME: SLEEP (HRS):

DATE _______________

NOTES FOR THE DAY

IN A STATE OF KETOSIS?

YES   NO   UNSURE

WATER INTAKE TRACKER

EXERCISE / WORKOUT ROUTINE

DAILY ENERGY LEVEL

HIGH   **MEDIUM**   **LOW**

BREAKFAST

FAT: CARBS: PROTEIN: CALORIES:

LUNCH

FAT: CARBS: PROTEIN: CALORIES:

DINNER

FAT: CARBS: PROTEIN: CALORIES:

SNACKS

FAT: CARBS: PROTEIN: CALORIES:

HOW DO I FEEL TODAY?

TOP 6 PRIORITIES OF THE DAY

END OF THE DAY TOTAL OVERVIEW

CARBS   FAT   PROTEIN   CALORIES

DAILY PROGRESS TRACKER

SLEEP TRACKER:

DATE

RISE:

BEDTIME:

SLEEP (HRS):

NOTES FOR THE DAY

IN A STATE OF KETOSIS?

YES   NO   UNSURE

WATER INTAKE TRACKER

EXERCISE / WORKOUT ROUTINE

DAILY ENERGY LEVEL

HIGH   MEDIUM   LOW

BREAKFAST

FAT: CARBS: PROTEIN: CALORIES:

LUNCH

FAT: CARBS: PROTEIN: CALORIES:

HOW DO I FEEL TODAY?

DINNER

FAT: CARBS: PROTEIN: CALORIES:

SNACKS

FAT: CARBS: PROTEIN: CALORIES:

TOP 6 PRIORITIES OF THE DAY

END OF THE DAY TOTAL OVERVIEW

CARBS   FAT   PROTEIN   CALORIES

DAILY PROGRESS TRACKER

SLEEP TRACKER:

DATE _______________

 RISE: ________

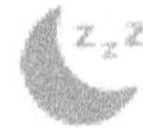 BEDTIME: ________

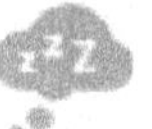 SLEEP (HRS): ________

NOTES FOR THE DAY

IN A STATE OF KETOSIS?

YES   NO   UNSURE

WATER INTAKE TRACKER

EXERCISE / WORKOUT ROUTINE

DAILY ENERGY LEVEL

HIGH   MEDIUM   LOW

BREAKFAST

FAT: CARBS: PROTEIN: CALORIES:

LUNCH

FAT: CARBS: PROTEIN: CALORIES:

DINNER

FAT: CARBS: PROTEIN: CALORIES:

SNACKS

FAT: CARBS: PROTEIN: CALORIES:

HOW DO I FEEL TODAY?

TOP 6 PRIORITIES OF THE DAY

END OF THE DAY TOTAL OVERVIEW

CARBS   FAT   PROTEIN   CALORIES

 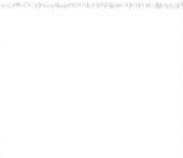 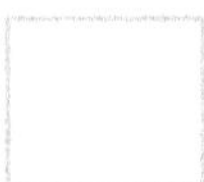 

DAILY PROGRESS TRACKER

SLEEP TRACKER:

DATE _______________

RISE: _______ BEDTIME: _______ SLEEP (HRS): _______

NOTES FOR THE DAY

IN A STATE OF KETOSIS?

YES   NO   UNSURE

WATER INTAKE TRACKER

EXERCISE / WORKOUT ROUTINE

DAILY ENERGY LEVEL

HIGH   MEDIUM   LOW

BREAKFAST

FAT: CARBS: PROTEIN: CALORIES:

LUNCH

FAT: CARBS: PROTEIN: CALORIES:

DINNER

FAT: CARBS: PROTEIN: CALORIES:

SNACKS

FAT: CARBS: PROTEIN: CALORIES:

HOW DO I FEEL TODAY?

TOP 6 PRIORITIES OF THE DAY

END OF THE DAY TOTAL OVERVIEW

CARBS   FAT   PROTEIN   CALORIES

DAILY PROGRESS TRACKER

SLEEP TRACKER:

DATE ____________

RISE:

BEDTIME:

SLEEP (HRS):

NOTES FOR THE DAY

IN A STATE OF KETOSIS?

YES　　　NO　　　UNSURE

WATER INTAKE TRACKER

EXERCISE / WORKOUT ROUTINE

DAILY ENERGY LEVEL

HIGH　　　MEDIUM　　　LOW

BREAKFAST

FAT:　CARBS:　PROTEIN:　CALORIES:

LUNCH

FAT:　CARBS:　PROTEIN:　CALORIES:

DINNER

FAT:　CARBS:　PROTEIN:　CALORIES:

SNACKS

FAT:　CARBS:　PROTEIN:　CALORIES:

HOW DO I FEEL TODAY?

TOP 6 PRIORITIES OF THE DAY

END OF THE DAY TOTAL OVERVIEW

CARBS　　　FAT　　　PROTEIN　　　CALORIES

WEEKLY FASTING TRACKER

Week Of: _______________

MONDAY

| Goal | 12 | 1 | 2 | 3 | 4 | 5 | 6 | 7 | 8 | 9 | 10 | 11 | 12 | 1 | 2 | 3 | 4 | 5 | 6 | 7 | 8 | 9 | 10 | 11 |
| Actual | 12 | 1 | 2 | 3 | 4 | 5 | 6 | 7 | 8 | 9 | 10 | 11 | 12 | 1 | 2 | 3 | 4 | 5 | 6 | 7 | 8 | 9 | 10 | 11 |

TUESDAY

| Goal | 12 | 1 | 2 | 3 | 4 | 5 | 6 | 7 | 8 | 9 | 10 | 11 | 12 | 1 | 2 | 3 | 4 | 5 | 6 | 7 | 8 | 9 | 10 | 11 |
| Actual | 12 | 1 | 2 | 3 | 4 | 5 | 6 | 7 | 8 | 9 | 10 | 11 | 12 | 1 | 2 | 3 | 4 | 5 | 6 | 7 | 8 | 9 | 10 | 11 |

WEDNESDAY

| Goal | 12 | 1 | 2 | 3 | 4 | 5 | 6 | 7 | 8 | 9 | 10 | 11 | 12 | 1 | 2 | 3 | 4 | 5 | 6 | 7 | 8 | 9 | 10 | 11 |
| Actual | 12 | 1 | 2 | 3 | 4 | 5 | 6 | 7 | 8 | 9 | 10 | 11 | 12 | 1 | 2 | 3 | 4 | 5 | 6 | 7 | 8 | 9 | 10 | 11 |

THURSDAY

| Goal | 12 | 1 | 2 | 3 | 4 | 5 | 6 | 7 | 8 | 9 | 10 | 11 | 12 | 1 | 2 | 3 | 4 | 5 | 6 | 7 | 8 | 9 | 10 | 11 |
| Actual | 12 | 1 | 2 | 3 | 4 | 5 | 6 | 7 | 8 | 9 | 10 | 11 | 12 | 1 | 2 | 3 | 4 | 5 | 6 | 7 | 8 | 9 | 10 | 11 |

FRIDAY

| Goal | 12 | 1 | 2 | 3 | 4 | 5 | 6 | 7 | 8 | 9 | 10 | 11 | 12 | 1 | 2 | 3 | 4 | 5 | 6 | 7 | 8 | 9 | 10 | 11 |
| Actual | 12 | 1 | 2 | 3 | 4 | 5 | 6 | 7 | 8 | 9 | 10 | 11 | 12 | 1 | 2 | 3 | 4 | 5 | 6 | 7 | 8 | 9 | 10 | 11 |

SATURDAY

| Goal | 12 | 1 | 2 | 3 | 4 | 5 | 6 | 7 | 8 | 9 | 10 | 11 | 12 | 1 | 2 | 3 | 4 | 5 | 6 | 7 | 8 | 9 | 10 | 11 |
| Actual | 12 | 1 | 2 | 3 | 4 | 5 | 6 | 7 | 8 | 9 | 10 | 11 | 12 | 1 | 2 | 3 | 4 | 5 | 6 | 7 | 8 | 9 | 10 | 11 |

SUNDAY

| Goal | 12 | 1 | 2 | 3 | 4 | 5 | 6 | 7 | 8 | 9 | 10 | 11 | 12 | 1 | 2 | 3 | 4 | 5 | 6 | 7 | 8 | 9 | 10 | 11 |
| Actual | 12 | 1 | 2 | 3 | 4 | 5 | 6 | 7 | 8 | 9 | 10 | 11 | 12 | 1 | 2 | 3 | 4 | 5 | 6 | 7 | 8 | 9 | 10 | 11 |

WEEKLY MEAL PLANNER

Week of:

	Breakfast	Lunch	Dinner	Snack	Other
Monday	TOTAL Carbs Fat Protein Cals	TOTAL Carbs Fat Protein Cals	TOTAL Carbs Fat Protein Cals	TOTAL Carbs Fat Protein Cals	TOTAL Carbs Fat Protein Cals
Tuesday	TOTAL Carbs Fat Protein Cals	TOTAL Carbs Fat Protein Cals	TOTAL Carbs Fat Protein Cals	TOTAL Carbs Fat Protein Cals	TOTAL Carbs Fat Protein Cals
Wednesday	TOTAL Carbs Fat Protein Cals	TOTAL Carbs Fat Protein Cals	TOTAL Carbs Fat Protein Cals	TOTAL Carbs Fat Protein Cals	TOTAL Carbs Fat Protein Cals
Thursday	TOTAL Carbs Fat Protein Cals	TOTAL Carbs Fat Protein Cals	TOTAL Carbs Fat Protein Cals	TOTAL Carbs Fat Protein Cals	TOTAL Carbs Fat Protein Cals
Friday	TOTAL Carbs Fat Protein Cals	TOTAL Carbs Fat Protein Cals	TOTAL Carbs Fat Protein Cals	TOTAL Carbs Fat Protein Cals	TOTAL Carbs Fat Protein Cals
Saturday	TOTAL Carbs Fat Protein Cals	TOTAL Carbs Fat Protein Cals	TOTAL Carbs Fat Protein Cals	TOTAL Carbs Fat Protein Cals	TOTAL Carbs Fat Protein Cals
Sunday	TOTAL Carbs Fat Protein Cals	TOTAL Carbs Fat Protein Cals	TOTAL Carbs Fat Protein Cals	TOTAL Carbs Fat Protein Cals	TOTAL Carbs Fat Protein Cals

WEEKLY LOW CARB SHOPPING LIST

FRESH PRODUCE

MEAT AND SEAFOOD

DAIRY PRODUCTS

PANTRY ITEMS

FROZEN / OTHER

DAILY PROGRESS TRACKER

SLEEP TRACKER:

DATE _______________

RISE: _______ BEDTIME: _______ SLEEP (HRS): _______

NOTES FOR THE DAY

____

____

____

IN A STATE OF KETOSIS?

YES   NO   UNSURE

WATER INTAKE TRACKER

EXERCISE / WORKOUT ROUTINE

DAILY ENERGY LEVEL

HIGH   MEDIUM   LOW

BREAKFAST

FAT: CARBS: PROTEIN: CALORIES:

LUNCH

FAT: CARBS: PROTEIN: CALORIES:

DINNER

FAT: CARBS: PROTEIN: CALORIES:

SNACKS

FAT: CARBS: PROTEIN: CALORIES:

HOW DO I FEEL TODAY?

TOP 6 PRIORITIES OF THE DAY

____

____

END OF THE DAY TOTAL OVERVIEW

CARBS   FAT   PROTEIN   CALORIES

DAILY PROGRESS TRACKER

SLEEP TRACKER:

DATE _______________

RISE: _______   BEDTIME: _______   SLEEP (HRS): _______

NOTES FOR THE DAY	IN A STATE OF KETOSIS?
	YES NO UNSURE

WATER INTAKE TRACKER

EXERCISE / WORKOUT ROUTINE

DAILY ENERGY LEVEL

HIGH   MEDIUM   LOW

BREAKFAST

FAT: CARBS: PROTEIN: CALORIES:

LUNCH

FAT: CARBS: PROTEIN: CALORIES:

HOW DO I FEEL TODAY?

DINNER

FAT: CARBS: PROTEIN: CALORIES:

SNACKS

FAT: CARBS: PROTEIN: CALORIES:

TOP 6 PRIORITIES OF THE DAY

END OF THE DAY TOTAL OVERVIEW

CARBS   FAT   PROTEIN   CALORIES

DAILY PROGRESS TRACKER

SLEEP TRACKER:

DATE

RISE: BEDTIME: SLEEP (HRS):

NOTES FOR THE DAY

IN A STATE OF KETOSIS?

YES   NO   UNSURE

WATER INTAKE TRACKER

EXERCISE / WORKOUT ROUTINE

DAILY ENERGY LEVEL

HIGH   MEDIUM   LOW

BREAKFAST

FAT: CARBS: PROTEIN: CALORIES:

LUNCH

FAT: CARBS: PROTEIN: CALORIES:

DINNER

FAT: CARBS: PROTEIN: CALORIES:

SNACKS

FAT: CARBS: PROTEIN: CALORIES:

HOW DO I FEEL TODAY?

TOP 6 PRIORITIES OF THE DAY

END OF THE DAY TOTAL OVERVIEW

CARBS   FAT   PROTEIN   CALORIES

DAILY PROGRESS TRACKER

SLEEP TRACKER:

DATE

RISE: BEDTIME: SLEEP (HRS):

NOTES FOR THE DAY

IN A STATE OF KETOSIS?

YES   NO   UNSURE

WATER INTAKE TRACKER

EXERCISE / WORKOUT ROUTINE

DAILY ENERGY LEVEL

HIGH   **MEDIUM**   **LOW**

BREAKFAST

FAT: CARBS: PROTEIN: CALORIES:

LUNCH

FAT: CARBS: PROTEIN: CALORIES:

HOW DO I FEEL TODAY?

DINNER

FAT: CARBS: PROTEIN: CALORIES:

SNACKS

FAT: CARBS: PROTEIN: CALORIES:

TOP 6 PRIORITIES OF THE DAY

END OF THE DAY TOTAL OVERVIEW

CARBS   FAT   PROTEIN   CALORIES

DAILY PROGRESS TRACKER

SLEEP TRACKER:

RISE: BEDTIME: SLEEP (HRS):

DATE

NOTES FOR THE DAY

IN A STATE OF KETOSIS?

YES   NO   UNSURE

WATER INTAKE TRACKER

EXERCISE / WORKOUT ROUTINE

DAILY ENERGY LEVEL

HIGH   MEDIUM   LOW

BREAKFAST

FAT: CARBS: PROTEIN: CALORIES:

LUNCH

FAT: CARBS: PROTEIN: CALORIES:

HOW DO I FEEL TODAY?

DINNER

FAT: CARBS: PROTEIN: CALORIES:

SNACKS

FAT: CARBS: PROTEIN: CALORIES:

TOP 6 PRIORITIES OF THE DAY

END OF THE DAY TOTAL OVERVIEW

CARBS   FAT   PROTEIN   CALORIES

DAILY PROGRESS TRACKER

SLEEP TRACKER:

DATE _______________

RISE: ____________   BEDTIME: ____________   SLEEP (HRS): ____________

NOTES FOR THE DAY

IN A STATE OF KETOSIS?

YES   NO   UNSURE

WATER INTAKE TRACKER

EXERCISE / WORKOUT ROUTINE

DAILY ENERGY LEVEL

HIGH   **MEDIUM**   **LOW**

BREAKFAST

FAT: CARBS: PROTEIN: CALORIES:

LUNCH

FAT: CARBS: PROTEIN: CALORIES:

HOW DO I FEEL TODAY?

DINNER

FAT: CARBS: PROTEIN: CALORIES:

SNACKS

FAT: CARBS: PROTEIN: CALORIES:

TOP 6 PRIORITIES OF THE DAY

END OF THE DAY TOTAL OVERVIEW

CARBS   FAT   PROTEIN   CALORIES

DAILY PROGRESS TRACKER

SLEEP TRACKER:

DATE

RISE: BEDTIME: SLEEP (HRS):

NOTES FOR THE DAY

IN A STATE OF KETOSIS?

YES   NO   UNSURE

WATER INTAKE TRACKER

EXERCISE / WORKOUT ROUTINE

DAILY ENERGY LEVEL

HIGH   **MEDIUM**   **LOW**

BREAKFAST

FAT: CARBS: PROTEIN: CALORIES:

LUNCH

FAT: CARBS: PROTEIN: CALORIES:

DINNER

FAT: CARBS: PROTEIN: CALORIES:

SNACKS

FAT: CARBS: PROTEIN: CALORIES:

HOW DO I FEEL TODAY?

TOP 6 PRIORITIES OF THE DAY

END OF THE DAY TOTAL OVERVIEW

CARBS   FAT   PROTEIN   CALORIES

MONTH THREE PROGRESS MEASUREMENTS

MONTHLY GOAL

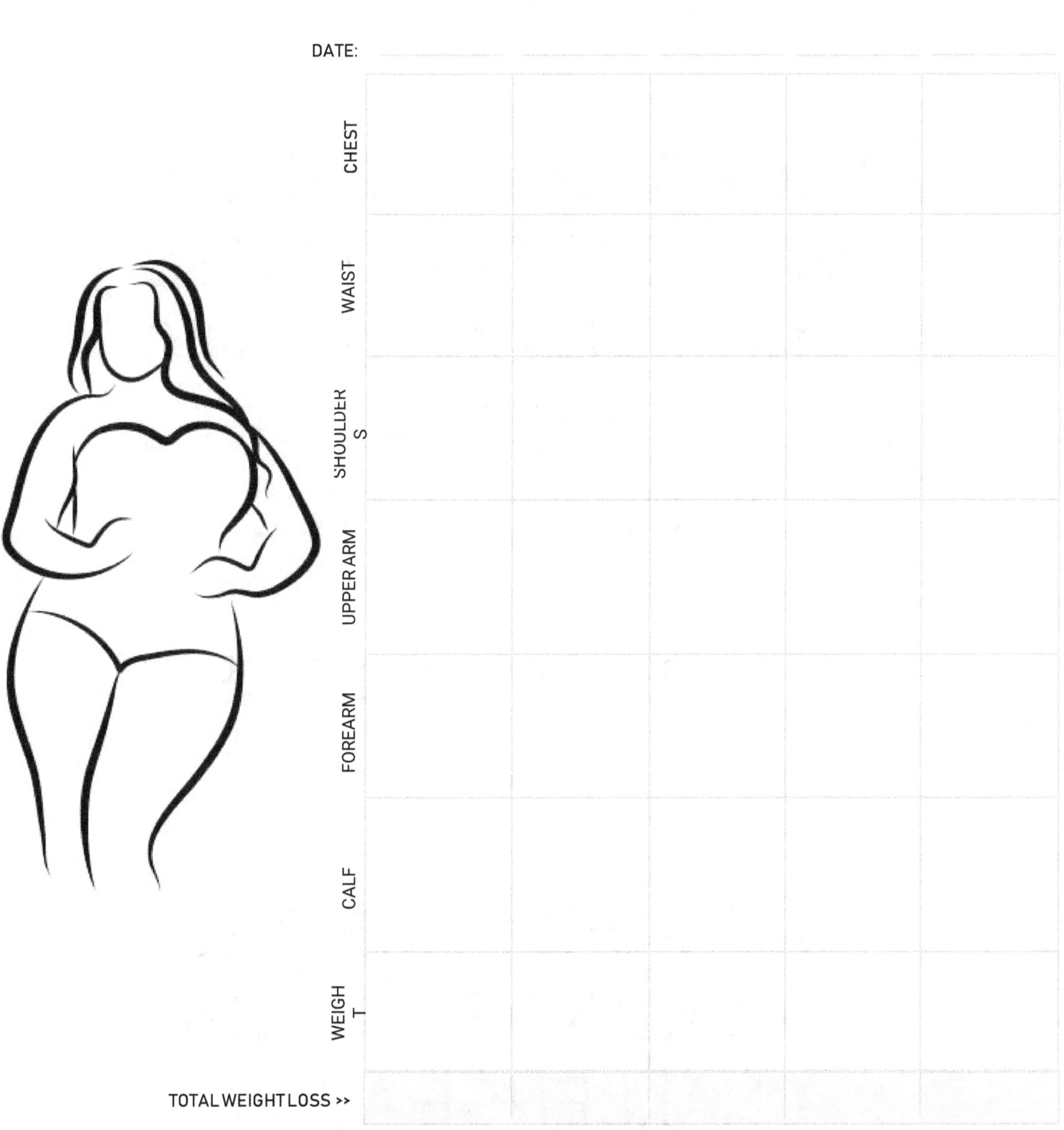

DATE:

CHEST

WAIST

SHOULDERS

UPPER ARM

FOREARM

CALF

WEIGHT

TOTAL WEIGHT LOSS >>

YOU DID IT.

YOU COMPLETED THE 90 DAY KETO CHALLENGE AND MADE KETOGENIC FOOD CHOICES A PART OF YOUR LIFESTYLE.

ARE YOU GOING TO KEEP IT UP?

RE-PURCHASE THIS BOOK AND START THE CHALLENGE AGAIN!

www.ingramcontent.com/pod-product-compliance
Lightning Source LLC
Chambersburg PA
CBHW081435250726
48662CB00009B/2800